DIABETES:
PREVENTION
AND CURE

DIABETES: PREVENTION AND CURE

C. Leigh Broadhurst, Ph.D.

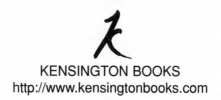

KENSINGTON BOOKS
http://www.kensingtonbooks.com

KENSINGTON BOOKS are published by

Kensington Publishing Corp.
850 Third Avenue
New York, NY 10022

ISBN 1-57566-471-2

First Printing: October, 1999
10 9 8 7 6 5 4 3 2

Printed in the United States of America

Contents

Introduction

The fundamental nutritional needs of humans have changed very little since the rise of our genus *Homo* 2–2.5 million years ago. Human nutritional requirements certainly have not changed significantly since the rise of our species *Homo sapiens* 100,000–300,000 years ago. Fully modern humans have been widespread for at least 40,000 years. These are long time spans compared to the 10,000 years since the initial adoption of agriculture, and the 50–100 years that modern processed foods have been available. For 99.8 percent of our time, we humans ate exclusively wild foods.

As far as human evolution is concerned, agriculture is a new experience—we are still in the initial stages of a grand experiment conducted on ourselves. We still have the bodies, metabolisms, and physiologies of Paleolithic hunter-gatherers. This means that the things that define what foods we need to build a healthy diet were determined thousands or millions of years ago, long before agriculture or even cooking was thought up. This simple, fundamental concept of our Paleolithic nature is usually glossed over, if even considered, by scientists and nonscientists alike. Convincing people that they are basically hunter-gatherers is often next to impossible—it just doesn't fit with our belief system.

Most of our major chronic diseases are brought upon us by straying from our evolutionary diet; that is, the diet naturally suited to our hunter-gatherer state of evolution. Problems occurred as soon as we adopted agriculture. And they have grown much worse in the processed food era, which began about 80 years ago.

The farther we stray from our evolutionary diet, the sicker

we become. The converse is true also: The sicker we become, the farther back in prehistory we have to go to pick foods that will heal us. Although major chronic diseases such as heart disease, cancer, stroke, and asthma are certainly related to our modern food choices, there is no better example of a disease brought upon us by straying from our Paleolithic diet than Type II diabetes, also called non-insulin-dependent diabetes mellitus (NIDDM) or adult-onset diabetes, because it usually occurs in people over 40 years old. Almost all diabetes—95 percent—is of this type.

Only 5 percent of diabetics have Type I diabetes, also known as insulin-dependent diabetes mellitus (IDDM) or juvenile diabetes. In Type I diabetes, the pancreas is dysfunctional and does not produce the hormone insulin. People with Type I diabetes need to inject insulin daily to remain alive, but they can certainly lower their insulin requirements, and dramatically improve their quality of life, by following a nutritional program.

People with Type II diabetes differ greatly in that they typically have adequate or even too much insulin, but this insulin is not utilized effectively. Insulin receptors on the cells may not "accept" insulin correctly, or perhaps the cells have fewer receptors than they should. In either case, the main result is that blood sugar (glucose) levels are both too high overall and poorly regulated. Since glucose is the primary fuel for the body, its regulation is crucial to our metabolisms. We simply can't function if insulin doesn't do its job. Insulin is primarily known for escorting glucose (a carbohydrate) to our cells, but it also escorts proteins and fats. This means that a diabetic's metabolic, growth, repair, and detoxification functions are *all* compromised *all* the time!

The bad news is that Type II diabetes is one of the biggest health problems in Western countries. It affects 6–12 million people in the United States alone, and the incidence is increasing despite continued advances in medical care. The good news is that Type II diabetes is first and foremost a nutritional disease—it is both caused and cured by appropriate nutrition. No one need suffer from this disease unless he or she chooses to do so. In this book, we will review the various nutritional causes of and effective nutritional treatments for Type II diabetes. These treatments are based on cutting-edge science, my years of personal consulting experience, and common sense. A number of the treatments can also be tailored to greatly help (but not cure) Type I diabetes, and specific instructions for Type I diabetics are given where appropriate. The treatments suggested here should not really be considered "alternative medicine." To the contrary, they are now or soon will be the treatments of choice for Type II diabetes.

While our bodies are still in the Stone Age, our culture and minds certainly are not. I use science to define what our real nutritional needs are, but I use practical common sense to design a diet that works for us today. The Modern Evolutionary Diet is designed to be as easy to follow as our current diet and lifestyles. The more diligently we follow this diet, the better and faster the results will be. But there is plenty of latitude (and even suggestions!) for cheating, because that's something we all need to do occasionally, regardless of whether it hinders our progress.

Type II diabetes is a nutritional disease that we have brought upon ourselves by our "experimentation" with agriculture. In my research, I have found that the major causes for Type II diabetes can all be related to a processed-food, agriculture-based diet. They are as follows:

- Obesity, or too much body fat with respect to the weight of lean tissue
- Too many calories, especially from refined and processed carbohydrates and fats
- Lack of certain polyunsaturated fatty acids and unbalanced fat intakes
- Chromium deficiency
- Lack of certain phytochemicals

Type II diabetes is a nutritional disease with a nutritional cure. The Modern Evolutionary Diet is the single best diet currently available for diabetics. In addition to the diet, there are supplements, herbs, and lifestyle changes that can truly help you, regardless of your ability to follow the diet closely. There is no reason why you or anyone you know who has Type II diabetes cannot control or completely reverse this condition. The dismal future for uncontrolled blood sugar includes blindness or vision impairment, irreversible nerve damage, kidney failure, heart disease, and early death. No drugs in the world can stop this progression, only slow it. Only you have the power to stop it.

I work at the Human Nutrition Research Center and the Environmental Chemistry Laboratories in a government research lab in Maryland. Researching chromium and fat nutrition and antidiabetic plants there, I've had the good fortune to work with one of the world's leading authorities on medicinal plants, Dr. James Duke, author of *The Green Pharmacy*.

I wrote this book to communicate the staggering truth that Type II diabetes is 99 percent a nutritional disease and can be treated nutritionally. The incidence of obesity and diabetes in Western countries keeps rising. So long as there is a 24-hour supply of cheap, abundant, tasty food, this incidence will continue to rise. Being told not to eat so much is not going to stop people. But if you know what foods to eat, what supplements you must have, and how to lose fat and gain muscle, *you* can prevent or reverse Type II diabetes naturally. You can also learn to control Type I diabetes naturally, and potentially prevent your infant from becoming diabetic if the condition runs in your family.

In this book, making the science understandable is one of my top priorities. Also, there's nothing recommended in this book that I haven't tried on myself and others. I've helped people with Type I, Type II, and gestational diabetes to control or reverse their condition. And I've helped hundreds of people adopt a diet through which they can lose body fat and, if they wish, gain muscle. I've also put my parents, grand-mother, and my husband's father and sisters on supplement plans that work for each of them. What I have to say can truly help people, provided they're ready to help themselves.

I've been an athlete all my life, particularly interested in weightlifting, swimming, and bicycling. I've tried everything from Tae Kwon Do to scuba diving. I'm married and have a 4½-year-old son and a 1½-year-old daughter. I do the cooking, food shopping, and serving. So when I make suggestions about how to get your family on a lifelong diet that will prevent obesity and diabetes, I'm talking in practical everyday terms.

Since the vast majority of diabetes cases are Type II, this is what our use of the word *diabetes* throughout the book refers to, unless otherwise stated.

The book is divided into three parts. The first part looks at the connection between nutrition and diabetes and at why so many Americans today are prone to diabetes. We see how the more we stray from our ancestral hunter-gatherer diet, the more likely we are to become diabetic. We examine how obesity can cause diabetes, and how exercise can help to control it. If you're obese and inactive, you can develop Type II diabetes before age 10. In fact, we're seeing huge increases in obesity-linked diabetes in children and young adults today. We also discuss the trace nutrient chromium as most effective against diabetes in one particular form. The first part closes by comparing essential structural fat and mostly nonessential storage fat.

The second part presents the Modern Evolutionary Diet. We learn here the basic guidelines to the diet, how to design meals, and how to maintain a desirable weight or even put on extra muscle (not fat). Chapter 9 gives practical advice on how to put the diet into everyday use, and a selection of recipes shows what to expect at the stove and the table.

The book's third part looks at natural cures and prevention. It's not widely known that food allergies are often associated with diabetes. Wheat products are frequently the allergens involved. Herbs, plant fiber, and even ground cinnamon have proven powers against diabetes. Other health problems associated with diabetes can be more troublesome than the condition itself. I offer natural remedies for the prevention and control of these complications.

Using the diet and recommendations contained in this book will go a long way toward granting a new lease on life to all diabetics. You can control Type I diabetes. And you can actually reverse Type II diabetes. This book shows you how to do it through safe and natural means. The rest is up to you!

PART
ONE

Nutrition and Diabetes

1

From Hunter-Gatherer to Diabetic Couch Potato

Most people think of agriculture as one of the greatest things that ever happened in the history of humankind. Indeed, chances are that neither you nor I would ever have been born if it were not for the great expansion of the population that agriculture allowed. However, the initial waves of population growth did not occur because the agricultural food supply was superior, but because people became sedentary, and could leave small children, the elderly, and the handicapped in the care of others. It is possible to see now that the population expansion occurred at great cost to our health and the health of the environment, and that perhaps we have let a genie out of a bottle that will never go back in.

The adoption of agriculture by hunter-gatherers was not a technological and lifestyle advancement, but was done only out of necessity. Adoption of agriculture initially resulted in *decreases* in human nutrition, health, and in some cases life-span. Hunting and gathering provides more calories, protein, and essential nutrients for a much smaller investment of time and energy expended than farming does.

What Hunter-Gatherers Ate

Archeologists and anthropologists have evaluated the composition of hunter-gatherer diets in prehistoric, historic, and existing populations. Preagricultural diets are now, and were in the past, exclusively dependent on animal protein and fat and wild vegetation. With the rare exception of honey, they never contained concentrated carbohydrate sources such as sugar, flour, rice, and pasta. In temperate and especially colder climates, carbohydrates were exceedingly limited. Traditional diets of Arctic societies can be virtually devoid of carbohydrate, consisting almost solely of animal protein and fat. Similarly, Northwest Coast Indians traditionally consumed great quantities of fatty fish. The fat was necessary for energy, because their carbohydrate sources were limited to clover roots that they occasionally dug up and wild berries collected during the short berry season.

Tropical and subtropical environments provided consistently higher amounts of carbohydrates in the form of fruits, honey, and starchy roots and tubers; however, fat- and protein-rich nuts often provided the largest percentage of calories from plant foods. Cereal grains were unknown, as were legumes such as soybeans and kidney beans. In some environments, legumes may have been consumed in their green state (like fresh peas or green beans). Dried mature beans were only occasionally utilized. Like cereal grains, mature legumes such as soybeans require organized agricultural production, and are also totally inedible unless cooked. In addition, many wild legumes are toxic.

Hunter-gatherers used game, fish, shellfish, birds, reptiles, amphibians, and insects for protein sources. Hunter-gatherers observed in historic times have been seen to waste nothing. Internal organs and brains of game are prized delicacies, consumed first and shared among the group due to their rich supply of essential nutrients. Fish brains and eyeballs are similarly prized, and a variety of frogs, lizards, snakes, and large insects are commonly roasted. In areas of Africa where wild honeybee hives are raided from time to time, the honeycomb is eaten with all the bee larvae intact. Nobody would be foolish enough to throw away this free source of protein and fat.

Robert Crayhon on Carbohydrates

The success of popular writer, lecturer, and talk-show host Robert Crayhon, M.S., is well deserved. If you need to get up to speed on general nutrition topics, read his books first! His explanations are clear, and his information is as correct as you're going to find. The following information can be found in more detail in his book *The Carnitine Miracle*. Crayhon told me: "Carbohydrates come in two varieties: paleocarbs, mainly fruits and vegetables—the kind we have eaten throughout our history; and neocarbs, those grain- and legume-based, refined carbohydrates that have surfaced in recent history. In Paleolithic times, virtually all our carbohydrates came from paleocarbs. Today in America, less than one-fourth of the carbohydrates we eat come from these foods. Most of the rest come from grain, grain products, and sugars. The worst part about the carbohydrate story is the creation of what I call 'ubiquifoods.' These are foods that are nearly omnipresent in our diet, to the point of causing nutritional and immunological insult. Examples of ubiquifoods include wheat, corn, dairy products, and soybeans. These are foods that all of us eat nearly every day, because they are shaped into many different processed foods.

"Wheat is a good example: We can easily eat wheat cereal or a muffin made from wheat for breakfast, a sandwich on wheat bread for lunch, and a dinner with wheat rolls or pasta. The body was never meant to eat the same food over and over again. But this can happen easily, thanks to the malleability of ubiquifoods and the wizardry of food processors. The result is food allergies, autoimmune diseases, and a lack of nutritional variation that can cause nutrient imbalances and deficiencies. Such ubiquifoods were never present in the Paleolithic diet, and a much greater variation of food sources exists in the wild. We

must follow our ancestors' example and eat a widely varied diet if our goal is optimal health.

"Since there are so many different ways of eating in the
wild, there is no single 'Paleolithic Diet.' There are many
different ways of eating, depending on where in the world
you are. But there are principles we can derive from the way
our ancestors ate that we can use to help us intelligently
hunt for food, as we walk down the danger-filled aisles of
the supermarket."

Fats in the Hunter-Gatherer Diet

On average, the total dietary fat in the hunter-gatherer diet
did not exceed 30–40 percent of total calories. However, their
diets were never fat-free, and some groups ate considerable
amounts of fat. They made great efforts to seek out and consume animal protein and fat. Edible fats were scarce, since
wild game is very lean compared to commercial livestock.
During the dry season in East Africa, for example, the fat content of hoofed game such as wildebeest and gazelle is only 1–4
percent by weight. This stands in contrast to the 20–30 percent fat by weight that is typical of meat from commercial livestock. Values higher than 30 percent fat are common in foods
such as cheese, bacon, and sausage.

In general, edible portions of wild game, fish, and shellfish
contain a *greater* percentage of structural fat and protein and
less storage fat per unit weight than does meat from livestock.
Structural fat is a major component of cell membranes, internal organs, and brain and nervous tissue. Structural fat contains a large proportion of polyunsaturated fatty acids, also
known as essential fatty acids (because they can't be manufactured by mammals and must be supplied from the diet).
Structural fat is also more roughly balanced in monounsaturated, polyunsaturated, and saturated fatty acids than storage
fat is.

For its part, *storage fat* has a higher proportion of saturated fatty acids, and sits in reserve or "storage" mainly on our hips, thighs, abdomens, and upper arms.

Storage fat served an important purpose for our ancestors. They needed to carry excess food with them, since food supplies were sporadic and unreliable, and people did not or could not store foods for any length of time. Other mammals also try to accumulate storage fat to get them through tough times. For example, white-tailed deer gorge on acorns in the fall to put on fat for winter. However, like our active ancestors, the deer use up this acorn fat (and more) to survive the winter and come spring, they are always lean and hungry. Our modern livestock are fed more than enough all the time and get very little exercise; so like modern humans, they gain lots of storage fat but use almost none of it.

Storage fat in animals, as in humans, has a higher percentage of saturated fatty acids. Meats with a good deal of marbling, for example, have both higher total amounts of fat, and higher relative amounts of saturated fatty acids per unit weight than do lean meats. This means that a pound of game meat or fish has much more protein, more essential fatty acids, and less saturated fat than a pound of typical grocery store meat does. This is especially true for beef, pork, and lamb as compared to buffalo, wild boar, and venison. It also means that most of the fat in game and fish is structural fat, and thus cannot be separated from the protein content when eaten. Our ancestors craved fat, but had to work for it—they simply didn't have rich fatty foods like cheese, bacon, and sausage, and didn't have separate sources of animal fat such as lard, butter, and duck fat.

Hunter-gatherers also consumed a seasonal variety of wild vegetables, fruits, seeds, and nuts. Fats in the vegetables, seeds, and nuts could not be separated from the protein, carbohydrate, and fiber contents. Just as there were no sugar, rice, and pasta, there were also no vegetable oils, peanut butter, chocolates, and refried beans. Our ancestors were probably excited to come across a tree full of ripe nuts, but they had plenty of competition from animals and birds. If no nuts or seeds were available, there was no handy store of olive oil or peanut butter to immediately satisfy their hunger for fat.

In other words, both animal and plant foods were consumed as whole unprocessed foods, and as a result, hunter-gatherers usually ate protein, fat, and carbohydrate together. If not, they ate mainly protein, because both carbohydrate and fat could be very scarce at times. What they did *not* eat was excessive amounts of carbohydrate and fat together. That combination is reserved for today's dietary specialties — including doughnuts, candy bars, fettuccini Alfredo, and potato chips.

Our ancestors also routinely ingested a whole array of vitamins, minerals, and beneficial phytochemicals. These nutrients were nothing short of obligatory for our ancestors—they had no means of preserving or processing foods, so that it was either eat fresh whole foods or starve. Nobody could decline fish brains and wild kale and, instead, send out for chicken wings and a large pizza, with a 2-liter Pepsi. The whole plant foods they ate, coupled with the lean protein, helped maintain normal blood glucose and insulin response. This combination is basically the best choice of foods to prevent diabetes.

Changes with Agriculture and Food Processing

The agricultural revolution changed the hunter-gatherer diet dramatically. Cereal grains became the basis for both human and livestock nutrition, and also the origin of the majority of our chronic diseases. Agriculture and modern food processing have led to averages of over 30 percent of total calories from fat in Western diets. Our diets also have a preponderance of saturated fatty acids and *trans*-fats, and often fewer polyunsaturated fatty acids than we need.

We also don't consume all our fat as a structural component of foods. Instead, we separate fat from whole foods, refine it, process it, and then *re-add* it to our foods! This re-addition typically increases the amount of fat in foods, while decreasing the amount of nutrients and phytochemicals (and often protein) that were obligatory for our ancestors. This same separation, refining, processing, and re-addition are also practiced on carbohydrate foods to an enormous extent. Sugar in one form or another is added to the majority of food products available in North American supermarkets. Although a diet composed of fresh-cut sugar cane, whole fruits, and cooked whole-grain porridge cannot be criticized too severely, the "Western standards" for carbohydrate consumption are based mainly on even worse foods: refined sugar, breads, pastries, desserts, and pastas made from white flour, fruit juices, and jellies. Under the current economic structure for food production and distribution, efforts to change this on a large scale will not be successful. Our society heavily discounts and promotes commodities such as sugar, corn syrup, wheat flour, processed cheese, and soybean oil, making them consistently cheaper and more readily available than fresh produce, meat, or fish.

A diet of mature dried cereal grains and legumes is a more dense source of calories than the natural diet of livestock and poultry, which naturally graze, scratch, and forage to find enough to eat. Foraging requires lots of energy to walk or fly around in search of food. It also takes a lot of energy to chew and digest grass and weeds. When livestock and poultry are confined to feedyards and cages, and fed rich grains, soybeans, peanuts, and various by-products from the oil-pressing industry, they gain lots of storage fat. We know that eating a diet rich in high-fat meats from intensively raised livestock is an important risk factor for chronic disease. In effect, we are transferring storage fat from one animal to another! Not as widely recognized but equally important, agriculture and food processing have led to imbalances in polyunsaturated fatty acid nutrition. These imbalances, in turn, promote the development of diabetes.

Obesity, abnormally high levels of insulin, and eventually diabetes are the natural consequences of successful agriculture. We have successfully achieved a chronic overabundance of food, while our bodies have retained a physiology that cannot handle chronic overeating.

In this book, I tell you what you need to know about the unhealthful foods of the modern world that have caused an epidemic of diabetes in America. I show you how to go about eating the healthful diet of our ancestors! My Modern Evolutionary Diet provides vitamins, minerals, and phytochemicals that approximate what our ancestors ate in the past.

What About Genetics?

While there is some genetic propensity for development of diabetes, the cause of this disease is largely nutritional. The small number of genetic factors currently identified with diabetes are likely to be activated by current Western diets. We have many genes, some known and even more unknown, that can influence our ability to develop a chronic disease or condition. In all but a minority of cases, our environment, diet, and lifestyle give our bodies signals that strongly affect whether these genes are activated or sit relatively idle. Although your risk for any disease may be higher if others in your family have had it, it does not mean you are *absolutely destined* to get it yourself. You can choose your diet and lifestyle to minimize your risk of diabetes, for example, and if your choices are good and you stick with them, their effect can more than compensate for your increased genetic risk. In other words, *you* make positive choices that prevent or minimize the expression of genes that cause abnormalities.

The incidence of diabetes among seven United States ethnic minorities for which there are data is much higher than the incidence in their respective countries of origin. When members of any ethnic group move to the United States, their incidence of diabetes increases. This is unequivocal evidence that Type II diabetes is caused by diet and lifestyle.

In the United States, the incidence of Type II diabetes is higher among non-Caucasians than Caucasians. In addition, genetic variation influences the incidence of diabetes among ethnic groups. This variation may suggest why ethnic groups that were among the first to adopt agriculture-based diets now have the lowest incidence of Type II diabetes.

The 50 percent overall incidence of diabetes in the Pima Indians of Arizona, however, is the highest of any ethnic group known. The Pima have been shown to have an intestinal protein gene type that allows protein to bind to fats more efficiently than in other people. This improved binding may help increase the absorption of fats in the intestine. This gene is also associated with higher average fasting glucose levels, and high insulin production in response to both glucose and mixed meals. But there is no consistent evidence to link this gene *directly* to diabetes. In many cases, the individuals in the genetic studies were already obese and insulin resistant, and so it can't be determined to what degree increased dietary fat availability or absorption is a nutritional or genetic influence on the development of diabetes.

If one or both of your parents are diabetic, you should consider yourself at increased risk for developing the disease and start following the suggestions in this book *before* you become diabetic. If you are a diabetic parent, don't let your children follow the same nutritional path that you have. Reversing your own disease is the best example you can ever set for them.

It is clear from research that there is no single "diabetes gene." Although whole families or even ethnic groups can have a tendency to develop diabetes, they almost always have a tendency to develop obesity also. Identical twins from ethnic groups prone to diabetes have a 70 percent chance of both developing the condition, but neither has to get it if they watch their diets.

It seems fairly certain that genes conferring a tendency to develop diabetes did not pose the same risk in the past as they do today in North America, Europe, and Australia. Diabetes is nearly nonexistent in some developing countries, and was not a major health problem in Western Europe during the lean years of World War II. Some genetic factors that lead to diabetes today may have been positive, life-preserving adaptations for Paleolithic humans. They are only rendered negative by straying from our evolutionary diet.

In certain select study populations, defects that significantly reduce insulin-controlled glucose uptake by skeletal muscles, glycogen synthesis and storage, insulin sensitivity, and insulin secretion have been found to be inheritable as well. The inheritance of these defects follows a simple non-sex-linked pattern known as autosomal, in which children of parents with the condition have a known chance of developing the same condition that can be statistically calculated. It has been shown, for example, that the offspring of two Type II diabetic parents become insulin resistant at a fairly young age, often years before they develop active diabetes. Defects in pancreatic beta-cell function and synthesis of the insulin molecule are also inherited. Although these autosomal patterns are observed, no genes that control the inheritance have been identified. A complex set of genes may exist that confers an inherited *susceptibility* to diabetes but does not actually *cause* the disease independent of nutritional and environmental factors.

Symptoms

Mark Swanson, N.D., of the Good Doctor, Inc., Neuropathic Wellness & Diagnosis Center, in Sequim, Washington, diagnoses diabetic patients holistically. Here he describes the health problems that eventually drive them to seek help:

"Most adult patients do not go to the doctor complaining of Type II diabetes," Dr. Swanson says. "Their initial complaint is rarely: 'I feel like my blood sugar is too high.' Instead, it's usually one or more of the following complaints: chronic fatigue, skin problems, poor digestion, aching joints, tender muscles, reduced immunity, depression, impotence, food cravings, inability to lose weight, chest discomfort, shortness of breath, high cholesterol, or high blood pressure. Diabetes is usually identified through a medical history, examination, and laboratory screening. These adults are usually (but not always) physically inactive and over their ideal body weight— they're the pot-belly crowd who eat a refined, processed diet, high in calories, simple carbohydrates, saturated fat, and *trans*-fatty acids, but low in fiber and essential fatty acids. Often, my patients have been previously diagnosed with diabetes and they come here because their diabetic diet doesn't work (most standard diabetic diets don't!) or their health has deteriorated due to the onset of diabetic complications. They've experienced first-hand the failure of the "recommended" American Diabetes Association Diet.

"My treatment goal is to correct *all* the disturbed biochemistry common to the condition of insulin resistance, of which overt diabetes is only one manifestation. Therefore, as a baseline, I treat all cases of insulin resistance the same whether they have diabetes or not. If you put your finger over the blood sugar reading on a typical laboratory chemistry profile, you can't tell the difference between the diabetic and nondiabetic person with insulin resistance. They both have cholesterol and lipid imbalances, high fasting insulin, and usually some elevation in glycated hemoglobin. I also look closely at uric acid, homocysteine, fibrinogen clotting factors, and C-reactive protein. C-reactive protein is a newly identified marker for low-level vascular wall inflammation leading to increased heart attack risk. Liver enzymes may be mildly elevated also.

"All diabetic patients are under increased oxidative stress throughout their bodies, especially in the heart blood vessels. These patients require additional antioxidant therapy and polyunsaturated fatty acids to keep cell membranes intact and lessen the micro-damage. I also see gross disturbances in intracellular electrolytes. This is observed clinically as low magnesium and/or potassium,

with a corresponding increase in calcium. On the digestive front, I see more irritable bowel syndrome, constipation, and bacterial and yeast overgrowth problems, as
well as increased intestinal permeability, in diabetic
patients. Functional liver testing often reveals an
impaired detoxification capacity. As you can see, diabetes and insulin resistance are reflections of a complex
interaction of disturbed biochemistry—a body out of
balance."

Blood Sugars and Hormones

All the carbohydrates that we eat are eventually broken
down to glucose (our bodies' primary fuel) and proteins and
fats that can be used to make glucose also. Blood sugar refers
to the concentration or level of glucose in the bloodstream.
Levels should never be too high or too low, and the body
operates normally when glucose concentrations are between
80 and 120 milligrams per deciliter. Since blood glucose levels
rise after eating, tests are usually done after fasting for 12
hours. If fasting levels are consistently high, this is an indica-
tion of possible diabetes.

Glycogen, the form in which glucose is stored by our liver and
muscles for energy, exists in amounts just enough to run the
body for less than a day. Our main source of stored energy is
fat. Glycogen is used for short bursts of intense activity, such as
lifting a very heavy weight or running 100 meters. Glycogen
was probably very useful for our ancestors when faced with
emergencies such as dangerous wounded game or a collapsing
cave roof. When glycogen is depleted by exercise or stress,
insulin helps build up the supplies as soon as food is eaten.

Glucose tolerance tests are used to spot individuals who may
be diabetic. In such a test, a standard glucose dose is admin-
istered, and the rise, peak, and fall of blood glucose is mon-
itored over the next few hours. If glucose is normally
metabolized or "tolerated," the resulting curve is normal.

Both the area under the curve and the peak are of interest. Blood sugar levels should not peak above certain values, and they should drop back to normal values after the test is complete. If glucose tolerance is poor, as is the case for diabetics, both the area under the curve and the peak value are abnormally large. This indicates that the individual has difficulty clearing glucose out of the blood. Tests can also be run in this fashion after a regular meal is consumed, instead of just glucose.

Insulin is a hormone secreted by the pancreas in response to rising blood sugar levels, such as after food is eaten and is beginning to be digested. Insulin escorts nutrients to cells, makes sure that the liver and muscle glycogen stores are filled up, and directs extra calories to be stored as fat.

Glucagon is insulin's partner hormone, and is secreted by the pancreas in response to falling blood sugar levels. Glucagon directs the liver to start using its glycogen stores to maintain blood sugar levels. It also mobilizes both fat *and* protein reserves for energy — unfortunately, high levels of glucagon don't burn only our body fat! Glucagon also stimulates us to seek food. Hormones such as epinephrine and cortisol are secreted when we are under stress, and work in conjunction with glucagon to mobilize fat and protein reserves. Chronically high levels of glucagon and these other hormones can cause severe hypoglycemia, muscle wasting, adrenal gland exhaustion, chronic fatigue, and liver dysfunction. As with all our hormonal systems, balance is the name of the game. Insulin and glucagon are both crucial to health, but neither should dominate.

Insulin sensitivity indicates how well tissues react to insulin. Type II diabetes is characterized by poor insulin sensitivity, meaning that tissues aren't responding to the hormone correctly or efficiently. These tissues may be described as being insulin resistant, indicating that their cells don't respond to insulin's signaling and don't take up nutrients from the bloodstream as well as they should. Insulin sensitivity can be estimated by keeping the blood sugar at a constant concentration with a steady glucose intake. Glucose is given slowly intravenously, for example, and the concentration of insulin in the bloodstream that the body must maintain in order to keep the blood sugar constant (that is, prevent it from rising precipitously) is measured. If the insulin concentration is significantly higher than normal, insulin sensitivity may be poorer than it should be.

Insulin sensitivity can also be estimated during glucose tolerance tests. Sometimes a person with poor insulin sensitivity may pass the glucose tolerance test, but the levels of insulin needed to pass the test are higher than normal. If the pancreas can keep producing this higher amount of insulin indefinitely, a person may not develop poor glucose tolerance or diabetes. However, if the high levels of circulating insulin cannot be maintained, as is typically the case, glucose tolerance gets progressively poorer, average blood sugar becomes increasingly elevated, and a person is on the road to diabetes.

Hyperglycemia is another word for high blood sugar.

Impaired or abnormal glucose metabolism is a condition in which the body is not capable of maintaining the tight regulation of blood sugar that good health requires. Impaired glucose metabolism may be caused by or associated with diabetes, but it can also be caused by medications, liver and kidney disease, adrenal gland dysfunction, cancer, candidiasis, obesity, and nutritional deficiencies.

Hypoglycemia or chronically low blood sugar also reflects abnormal glucose metabolism. However, hypoglycemia is *not* the reverse of diabetes. It is rarely a disease, merely a symptom—very often of undiagnosed food allergies, chronic consumption of sugar and wheat flour, candidiasis, thyroid gland dysfunction, or parasitic infections.

If you do not yet have diabetes but are concerned about it, you need never become diabetic if you heed the advice in this book. You will need to first understand the hunter-gatherer diet, and then start shifting your diet backward in time. If you are now diabetic, you *can* reverse your disease. You will just have to travel a little farther back in time, and spend a little longer visiting there than someone who is not. In both cases, a great number of vitamins, trace elements, and herbs can help make your trip faster and easier.

So, let's begin to take the trip back together.

2

Obesity and Diabetes

Obesity is unquestionably the major cause of Type II diabetes. If you are diabetic and overweight, you have almost certainly already been told by your doctor to drop some pounds. In many cases, a weight loss of 20–50 pounds is all that it takes to control or significantly improve diabetes. While the incidence of diabetes is already very high, millions more people have the disease and don't know it. This is especially true of fairly overweight or obese people over age 40. As the months or years pass, their glucose tolerance gets progressively poorer. They may not feel quite themselves, but perhaps attribute this malaise to the general effects of aging or obesity. Unfortunately, a diagnosis of diabetes is often not made until a person develops serious complications such as kidney disease, vision impairment, neurological or skin problems, or severe fluid retention in the legs and feet. Fortunately, doctors are increasingly performing routine screening for diabetes in patients who are liable to be at risk. A major incentive for more screening is the cost of diabetes to Medicare alone: $42.5 billion in 1995 and still increasing.

The relationship between diabetes and obesity is complex, and is best described by a feedback loop system. In a feedback loop system, when A affects B, B changes a little, and then B in turn affects A. The feedback loop is then repeated, with A affecting B, and B affecting A, and neither A nor B remaining exactly the same in each cycle. In the obesity-diabetes feedback loop, obesity (A) directly initiates diabetes (B), and once someone becomes diabetic to some degree, the new diabetic condition (changed B) causes obesity or makes it harder to lose weight, even if one is trying (changed A).

Obesity itself interferes with normal glucose metabolism, and decreases insulin sensitivity. In addition, insulin receptors on the cells that store fat don't seem to work as well when the cells are "stuffed" with storage fat. Conversely, chronically elevated levels of insulin can make fat loss more difficult and may increase appetite. Further, people with diabetes are often very sedentary, rarely if ever exercising strenuously. As diabetes worsens, some of the neurological and circulatory complications can strongly reduce your ability to get around and virtually prohibit exercise. The feedback system actually progresses in a downward spiral, which begins when you gain more than 20 pounds or so of excess fat. Aging, poor dietary choices, and nutritional deficiencies also contribute significantly to your downward slide. Certainly the best time to act is *before* you gain any more fat, and *before* you become diabetic. Otherwise, you're already in the feedback system, and every time your weight goes up 5 pounds or so, you're beginning another cycle of the feedback loop. You're spiraling down, increasing the severity of your diabetes, and increasing the likelihood that your weight loss efforts will not be rewarded by easy or rapid success.

In order to stay out of the sinking spiral leading to diabetes, your number one task is to maintain normal body weight through a healthful diet and regular exercise. If you are already a diabetic, you must also lose fat and exercise, but at the same time you should implement the many suggestions given in the following chapters in order to more quickly and successfully reverse the direction of the spiral. If you have diabetes but aren't overweight, exercising and following the suggestions are the most important tasks for you.

Now if you are overweight, your primary task is to start on a diet plan that will help you lose fat and do the best job possible of managing or preventing diabetes. It must be a diet plan that you can stick with, not a fad, gimmick, or an expensive proposition with a lot of premade, processed, specialty microwave meals. The Modern Evolutionary Diet for fat loss can do this job for you and more. Since our modern agriculture and processed food diet is almost wholly responsible for diabetes, readopting our evolutionary diet, to the best of our abilities, is far and away the most powerful tool we have to free ourselves of diabetes.

Overweight Means Overfat

It's very important to realize that the weight you need to lose to help control your diabetes is *fat*. A 300-pound bodybuilder doesn't have diabetes, because his weight comes from extra muscle, not extra fat. Muscles are active tissue and burn calories 24 hours a day. Your skeletal muscles are those that support your body, such as those found in legs, back, and arms. Skeletal muscles are by far the biggest users of glucose in your body. This means that the more muscles you have, and the more you use them, the lower your risk for developing diabetes. If you have a lot of muscles but also a lot of fat, such as some football defensive linemen, for example, this is better than just being fat, but still not the best you can do.

What's *really* important is having a high ratio of lean to fat tissue in your total body weight. A high ratio of lean to fat tissue is associated with a strongly decreased risk for diabetes. Lean tissue includes muscles, bones, tendons, ligaments, cartilage, and essential organs. A 300-pound bodybuilder is an extreme example, but serves the purpose well. On his body you can see every muscle, because his body fat level is only about 5–7 percent of his total body weight. He also has large, strong bones. He wants to gain and maintain muscle mass without gaining fat. Instead of being concerned about diabetes, he is concerned about having *low* blood sugar during intense workouts. Sometimes bodybuilders who do not have diabetes inject themselves purposely (and illegally) with extra insulin to help build muscle during workouts. This is dangerous, because it can cause exceedingly low blood sugar levels and even a "diabetic coma" from insulin overload. The important point here is that for diabetes, as well as virtually all other chronic diseases, lean body weight is your ally and fat is your enemy. Losing weight in the Modern Evolutionary Diet means losing *fat* and maintaining or gaining *muscle*.

The ratio of lean to fat tissue is important, even if you don't appear to be overweight. There is a very big difference between being lean and being skinny. Being lean means simply having a high ratio of lean to fat tissue. One may be lithe and wiry, or a 185-pound Ms. Universe contestant, but the bottom line is that a person needs a good muscular structure and a strong skeleton. Being skinny means that you don't have too much body fat, but you don't have too much muscle either! Skinny people have a lean to fat ratio that is either average, or in some cases below average. Below average lean to fat ratios are a common occurrence among dieters who eat too little protein and either don't exercise or like to run or jump about in aerobic dance classes. Being skinny may be preferable to being overfat or obese, but it does not protect you from diabetes as much as being lean does. Neither does it protect you from looking old before your time.

As we age, we tend naturally to lose muscle mass and, to a lesser degree, bone mass. We all know how different a man of 35 looks compared to a man of 75, even if their body weights are virtually the same. Older people often end up with very skinny arms and legs, and a large pot belly. Even if they don't have a large abdomen and are not considered "fat," the slow but steady loss of muscle and bone shifts the ratio of lean to fat tissue away from lean and toward fat. This is one reason why Type II diabetes is called adult-onset diabetes, and one of the factors responsible for the general trend of decreasing glucose tolerance with age.

Think about what signifies youth. Although a person may have a few wrinkles or gray hair, if that person has an *even distribution of body mass,* he or she does not look old. Once we allow ourselves to have a great big midsection and skinny arms and legs, *we look old!* What's more, we feel old, because it gets harder and harder for those weak arms and legs to carry us through our daily activities. Never mind how much you weigh, eat, or jump around in aerobics class—everyone should strive to have their shoulders broader than their hips until they die. There is no harm in having your vanity help you strive for this goal as much as your desire to prevent diabetes and other chronic diseases.

Central Obesity

Central obesity is a special kind of obesity that poses a greater-than-average risk to our health. Centrally obese people have a concentration of fat in the abdomen, chest, and upper arms, but may not have fat hips or legs. They are sometimes described as apple-shaped, and to a large degree a tendency to develop this condition appears to be genetic. Central obesity is associated with a high incidence of diabetes, as well as cardiovascular disease, high blood pressure, and premature death. In contrast, more normal distributions of fat are either spread underneath the skin all over or concentrated on the hips and thighs. A good deal of fat on the hips and thighs results in a pear-shaped body, which might be deemed unattractive but is not associated with the same risk for chronic disease as central obesity is.

Centrally obese individuals tend to have a diminished capability to use glucose in their skeletal muscles, skin, and bones. They also tend to have fewer insulin receptors on cells and have higher levels of free fatty acids and triglycerides in their bloodstreams. These higher blood levels of fat give the body a signal that lots of fat is available for energy. Hence glucose is not used as effectively, causing possibly higher-than-normal levels of glucose in the bloodstream.

How Did We Get So Fat?

Under our present circumstances in North America (especially) and Western Europe, the war against obesity can never be won. Virtually all human evolution was complete prior to the agricultural revolution. We are not even really designed to eat cooked food, let alone highly refined and processed foods like sugar, biscuits, and rice cakes. North Americans vastly overconsume sugars, grain products, *trans*-fatty acids, and animal fats, and underconsume fruits, vegetables, very lean meat, and seafoods. The combination of these factors is responsible for most obesity and chronic disease. Processed grains, sugars, and oils are unnatural to our ancient body and give us biochemical signals to overeat and eat often. Junk food diets are so nutrient-poor that they *require* the overconsumption of calories. You cannot fool your ancient body, and it will continue to signal for eating if the nutrients it requires are not provided. If the food you are eating is very nutrient-poor (white rice and doughnuts are good examples), you have no choice other than to eat a *lot* of calories to get your basic needs. And it doesn't help matters much to have inexpensive junk food readily available 24 hours a day, 7 days a week.

The Modern Evolutionary Diet for obesity and diabetes avoids extra carbohydrates and all refined, high-density carbohydrates. Many people who have successfully cut out fat in their diet lose weight quickly, and then plateau. Others cut out fat but still get nowhere. In both cases, this usually stems from a combination of poor nutrition, inactivity, and too much emphasis on carbohydrates. High intakes of fat do tend to make us fat. High intakes of carbohydrate don't always make us gain, but they can be very good at sparing existing fat, making it hard to lose weight. In effect, we never let our metabolism dip into the fat reserve bank, because the carbohydrate income is so steady. The more refined these carbohydrates, the worse the problem. Sugar and all pastries, cookies, cakes, and similar items are the worst, and pasta is second. Pasta is not a health food! In terms of nutrition content, it is a refined wheat product virtually identical to white bread—differing only in that it is eaten in even greater excess. These high-density dried grain carbohydrate foods are unnatural to our metabolisms, cause overeating, and are a major factor for development of diabetes.

If you are a sugar, pastry, or starchy food addict, this is the main source of your weight problem and must be resolved in order for you to take off fat and keep it off. If you eat two doughnuts with your morning coffee, you get 500 calories, but you do *not* get the protein, vitamins, trace elements, and essential fatty acids you need to function that morning. You may even be pumping up your energy level artificially with caffeine from the coffee, instead of from a healthful breakfast. In fact, doughnuts are so devoid of nutrients, they don't even contain enough vitamins and minerals to metabolize the calories they contain, so that your body must "cannibalize" or borrow nutrients from somewhere else. If you typically eat a healthful diet and take supplements, and this is just a random treat, no big deal. But if you are a pastry addict, remember that high-sugar, high-carbohydrate junk food diets lead directly to fatigue, obesity, and diabetes.

Strength Training

Bruce De Carlo, M.D., of the National Rehabilitation Hospital in Washington, D.C., is a specialist in physical medicine and rehabilitation. He is dedicated to strength training through lifting weights, which he says is highly beneficial for many rehabilitation patients, especially the elderly.

"Many of my patients need rehabilitation treatment for a long time," Dr. De Carlo said. "They often say that they would prefer to use a nutritional route for rehab, and many ask me questions about what vitamins and minerals they can take. Unfortunately, at the hospital, I can't prescribe supplements for them, but I do use supplements myself, and I can and do make suggestions to them and their family members as to how they can help speed their recovery."

Dr. De Carlo advocates a high-protein diet for himself and most of his patients. "Severe injuries, coupled with the effects of the stress hormones secreted during prolonged recovery, put people in a catabolic [muscle-wasting] state. They burn up their muscle and joint tissue, which weakens them and makes recovery even slower and less complete. I try to make sure their hospital meals are high in protein. Many of the nutrition principles and practices that bodybuilders use to gain lean body mass are directly applicable to these patients, and I wish more doctors understood that. After they leave the hospital, I talk to the patients and their family members about the importance of weight training for recovery, high-protein nutritious diets, and supplements."

Don't Be Gulled by the Glycemic Index

The glycemic index of carbohydrates has become a buzzword in the health food industry. People are told that they shouldn't eat foods such as carrots, corn, honey, potatoes, lima beans, beets, parsnips, turnips, bananas, raisins, and oranges, because they are high on the glycemic index.

Let's consider the carrot. Reading labels tells us that carrots don't have many calories per unit weight. Common sense tells us that (1) our ancestors ate lots of root vegetables, (2) carrot sticks are often used in successful diet plans, and (3) people who became diabetic by eating a big bowl of peas and carrots daily just don't exist. But nutritional scientists rate carrots at a whopping 92 or even much more out of a possible 100 on the glycemic index. Does this mean that carrots are a poor choice for diabetics? Let's find out.

The glycemic index is based on a 50-gram portion of carbohydrates provided by a food, or is based on eating the 50 grams of isolated digestible carbohydrate (that is, a pure sugar). It is *not* based on 50 grams of food per se, but rather the weight of food that is required to provide 50 grams of digestible carbohydrates. This means that the glycemic index does not necessarily compare foods on a reasonable serving-by-serving basis. It must be kept in mind that regardless of the glycemic index value, fresh vegetables and fruits, such as corn, peas, oranges, and carrots, are about 90 percent water. No matter how you slice it, produce is a very dilute source of carbohydrates compared to dried grains, beans, flour, and sugar. In fact, in one study, since nobody could eat the amount of carrots, turnips, broad beans, beets, or parsnips required to get 50 grams of carbohydrate, only 25-gram carbohydrate portions were used.

Remember that 100 grams of sugar has 100 grams of carbohydrate, but 100 grams of carrots has only 4.8 grams of carbohydrates. If you want to get 25 grams of carbohydrates from carrots, you need to eat 520 grams (1.2 pounds) of carrots! This is quite a lot of carrots at one sitting, and the energy burned chewing and digesting these carrots is not insignificant; neither is the large amount of fiber provided by the carrots.

In a 1994 study, 100-, 200-, and 300-gram portions of boiled carrots were fed to ten healthy men as part of a balanced meal. Creamed potatoes, jam, white bread, and light beer were provided as carbohydrate sources. After eating, the subjects were given a glucose tolerance test. It was found that the *larger* the carrot portion, the *lower* the glucose and insulin levels. This means that they did better on the glucose tolerance test when they ate carrots! The 200- and 300-gram portions were effective in lowering the peak glucose levels, too. The effects of the fiber, water, and phytochemicals in carrots far outweighed their minor carbohydrate contribution.

The glycemic index has great value in helping people choose unrefined foods over refined foods, but is not terribly important for preventing or reversing diabetes. Our ancestors only had fruits, vegetables, and some unrefined wild seeds and nuts to provide carbohydrates. They had no cereal grains, dried beans, flour, fruit juice, or sugar to apply a glycemic index to, and had no reason to worry about one. If you choose evolutionary foods and evolutionary eating principles, you don't have to do much worrying about the glycemic index either.

We're Designed for Starvation, Not Abundance

When food was plentiful for hunter-gatherers, feasting occurred over a short period of time—eating literally went on until the food was gone, and after a long rest, it was time to go out and find some more. The evolutionary purpose for overeating *is* to gain weight, and to a greater or lesser degree, we are all adapted to do so, or we would never have survived in the past. In the past, our storage fat was a life preserver ring around our waist rather than the spare tire of today.

A tendency to store fat and release insulin, as opposed to glucagon, was likely a positive factor for humans adapted to the evolutionary hunter-gatherer diet, but is maladaptive today. This is an adaptation to a diet (1) low in fat and often in calories, (2) raw and unprocessed, and (3) free from high-density carbohydrates. Unfortunately, and as we have seen, obesity, high insulin levels, and glucose intolerance are the natural consequences of successful agriculture. Yes, we have successfully achieved a chronic overabundance of food, while retaining a physiology that cannot handle chronic overeating!

Many aspects of our culture are designed more for starvation than for abundance. We attach huge significance to sharing meals, preparing delicious foods, and offering gifts of food to family, friends, and neighbors. We celebrate holidays with feasting and special rich foods. If you allow yourself to be riddled with guilt over others' expectations of your eating habits, you will have difficulty following the Modern Evolutionary Diet (or any diet, for that matter) and are bound to fail. This is not a book about diet psychology or personal motivation. Plenty of these books are available and evidently haven't had much impact. However, since your health is at stake, we do need to identify some common cultural pitfalls.

Good nutrition concerns not only the food you eat, but also the way you eat your food. Do you enjoy meal time or do you simply satisfy your hunger? Do you rush eating or do you take a special time for a special activity? Do you eat your lunch at a conference table or do business during your lunch? Perhaps without even realizing it, do you feed your children or family too much so that you can clean up their plates? Does stress make you reach for food?

While working on your goal of preventing or reversing diabetes, you may need to rethink your eating habits. Consider that the *way* you eat may tend to make you eat more food than is really required by your body. Good eating habits are also in tune with your digestive tract and better nutrient absorption. This starts with relaxing at meal time, eating slowly, and chewing your food well. Play a psychological game with yourself, and make a smaller quantity of food last longer than the larger quantity that you used to consume. Sipping water between bites can help this process.

Don't eat what people throw together for you, if you can't identify what's in it. As you improve your health, people will become jealous of you and will try to tempt you and thwart your efforts. Just politely decline. Setting a good example is the best defense (and offense) you could ever have, and is the only way to get the unwilling to eventually follow your lead. Similarly, at parties and holidays, where others are in charge of meals, eat heartily of the foods that fit your diet and make a point to praise them highly. Then you have plenty of ammunition to decline other foods without causing any bad feelings between you and your host or hostess. Don't be afraid to tell your host or hostess that you are working to prevent or reverse diabetes. If you are firm but discreet, you can use your disease as a dinner party crutch as often as you need to.

Try to avoid fast-food restaurants and old haunts where family and friends will encourage you to eat poorly, just because they are doing so themselves. Celebrate and enjoy eating with your family in a relaxed environment. Separate eating from watching TV, talking on the phone, or reading, if these distractions trigger you to eat too fast or too much. Eat more slowly, serve yourself smaller portions, and wait 20 minutes after eating your first serving before taking a second serving. Run some errands or go out for a walk after eating a satisfying meal, in order to avoid after-meal snacking or cleaning up plates. Pay your kids to do the dishes, so that you don't eat leftovers as you clean up. Brushing your teeth immediately after finishing a meal can keep you from continuing to eat or immediately reaching for a snack.

Type II Diabetes in Children?

Although Type II diabetes is primarily a disease of older people, our epidemic level of obesity in children and young adults is changing this situation. More and more young people are developing Type II diabetes as a consequence of eating too much junk food and exercising too little. Children younger than 10 years are showing up at doctors' offices with blood sugar many times higher than it should be. This is such a grave situation for our nation's health that the *New York Times* did a story on juvenile Type II diabetes on December 14, 1998. A Columbia University doctor interviewed in the story said that Type II diabetes was diagnosed in 10–20 percent of new pediatric cases in the university hospital's clinics, up from less than 4 percent five years ago. By the time these children are in their twenties, they have complications usually seen in people ages 60–70.

What all these children have in common is that they

are more than 20 percent over their ideal weight. They eat large quantities of high-carbohydrate, high-fat snacks, and spend long hours watching TV, playing video games, or sitting in front of a computer. They may watch and idolize their favorite basketball players, but unfortunately don't aspire to emulate the players' lean, fit bodies. A sad point about the article is that another doctor interviewed from the Juvenile Diabetes Foundation characterized these children as "people who would likely develop diabetes sometime during their lifetime, it's just that childhood obesity has brought it out earlier." In this book we *don't* consider Type II diabetes as a "fait accompli"—this is a nutritional disease with a nutritional cure, and in all but a handful of cases, it's completely preventable. Ask your grandmother how many kids had Type II diabetes in her elementary school!

Eight Changes in Our Diet That Cause Diabetes

Eight major differences exist between our diet and that of our hunter-gatherer ancestors. What we eat has changed, but not our bodies. Here are the eight differences and some of the consequences.

1. Refined and processed foods are now a huge part of our diet. The first and worst offender is refined grains. The obvious cases are white flour and white bread. However, most people don't realize that pasta, cream of wheat, pearled barley, most cereals, rice cakes, degerminated corn meal, and white rice are refined starches. The second worst offenders are the refined sugar and corn syrup included in sodas, candy, desserts, most commercial baked goods and cereals, many sauces, dips, and salad dressings. Foods such as candy, doughnuts, pastries, and store-bought cookies and cakes are to be avoided in any weight loss diet—even the new fat-free and low-fat versions. A high-sugar diet defeats

all attempts at fat loss. The third worst offenders are the hydrogenated and other *trans*-fats found in nearly all commercial baked and snack goods, deep-fried foods, and supermarket vegetable oils.

2. Our diet is too high in total fat, but too low in polyunsaturated fats, especially omega-3 fatty acids. A diet with 20 percent of its calories from fat that also includes balanced polyunsaturated fatty acid supplementation provides for successful body fat loss.

3. Protein intake is chronically too low. Contrary to what some claim, healthy humans are adapted to high-protein diets, and these provide excellent blood sugar control. High-protein snacks and meals make us feel full longer and with less food. Grains and beans have only minimal levels of protein.

4. Carbohydrate intake is chronically too high, especially in refined and processed forms from cereal grain products and sugars.

5. Diets with only 10 percent of total calories from fat are completely unnecessary for fat loss, and are hard to stick to. Fat-free foods do not satisfy persistent hunger. A little fat goes a long way to keep the stomach quiet! Moderation is the key here.

6. There's an extreme lack of fresh whole fruits, vegetables, and soluble fiber in our diet. Also, there's a general lack of vitamin C, magnesium, and phytochemicals as compared to hunter-gatherer diets.

7. We often eat soups, stews, casseroles, and slow-cooked foods. We also like canned, heavily salted, smoked, or preserved foods such as applesauce, pickles, cheeses, and deli-style meats. The more plain, fresh, raw food or lightly cooked food we consume, the better. Split pea soup, Irish stew, and cold cut subs were not our ancestors' style. They ate it fresh or not at all.

8. We no longer drink water exclusively, but very often sweet drinks or alcoholic drinks that use as much water to digest as they provide. Help yourself lose fat and pre-

vent disease by sipping plain water all day. It's great if you have to urinate at least every two hours while you're awake. The work time spent in the bathroom will pay you back more than double by increased alertness. Many of us are walking around constantly in a state of mild dehydration, and concentration on a task is the first to go.

3

Exercise Directly Improves Diabetes

Both anaerobic and aerobic exercises are beneficial for diabetes. Anaerobic or strength training refers almost exclusively to regular weightlifting, but may also include certain calisthenics and martial arts, wrestling, and rock climbing. The main purposes and benefits of anaerobic exercise are an increase in size and strength of the skeletal muscles. During anaerobic exercise the body usually does not move very far from a fixed position during the whole exercise session. Our metabolic rate may increase greatly while we are actually lifting a weight up and down, for example, but this huge increase is typically not sustained for more than a few minutes.

Aerobic exercise or cardiovascular training refers to exercise that significantly increases the speed at which the body moves, for example, running, swimming, dancing, skiing, and bicycling. In order to move the body faster, the rates of our metabolic functions such as heartbeat, respiration, and circulation must all increase. The primary purposes and benefits of aerobic exercise are a sustained increase in our metabolic rate, a stronger heart and circulatory system, and increased endurance. Muscles may become more toned, but do not necessarily become much stronger, and may actually decrease in size. During aerobic exercise, the body usually moves quite a distance from the starting point. Although exercise machines like stationary bikes and stair climbers keep us in a fixed place, they also keep track of how far we would have gone if we were let loose, so the principle is the same.

Exercise and Glucose Metabolism

Both anaerobic and aerobic exercise can permanently improve glucose metabolism. Some of the reasons for this improvement are as follows:

1. Exercise increases the metabolic rate, and with this increase, insulin receptors on the muscle cells are activated. Glucose uptake is greatly enhanced over sedentary levels.
2. With regular exercise training, the body adapts to the training condition and uses insulin more efficiently.
3. Regular exercise can increase insulin binding and insulin receptor number, thus improving the uptake of glucose, regardless of whether the body is exercising or at rest.
4. Regular exercise helps us lose body fat, and helps prevent us from gaining it back. Even more importantly, strength training can significantly increase the lean to fat body mass ratio. As we have discussed above, attaining a high lean to fat ratio is a major factor for preventing and reversing diabetes.
5. Exercise can lower total and LDL cholesterol levels, decrease blood pressure, and improve circulation, all of which help reverse or control diabetes and diabetic complications.

Regular exercise, at least 3 times a week for 30 minutes each time, does improve your metabolism, but does little to cause fat loss without dieting as well. Any kind of exercise is better than none, but meaningful, rigorous exercise increases health and strength more than "recreational" exercise. Exercise promotes weight loss, improves glucose tolerance in both Type I and II diabetics, lowers total serum cholesterol, increases HDL ("good") cholesterol, reduces blood pressure, prevents osteoporosis and hip fracture, and reduces constipation. Exercise also lowers the risk of stroke, cardiovascular disease, and certain types of cancer. It can slow down the aging process, and help prevent the significant loss of strength, balance, and coordination so often seen in the elderly. The most successful weight loss plans use a combination of diet and exercise. Exercise is also of great help in combating depression. In cases of depression or chronic bad moods, as little as one exercise session can lift the spirits and improve the mood.

If you have Type I diabetes, exercise cannot reverse your condition, but it can permanently lower your insulin requirements and slow the development of diabetic complications. Please consult your physician before you start on a rigorous program, because you will need to carefully monitor your blood sugar before and after you exercise. If you have been sedentary, start out exercising for no more than 30 minutes at a time, and perform the exercise at a place and time where it is easy for you to monitor your health. Don't, for example, travel a long distance to a new health club or exercise right before bedtime. As you slowly increase the frequency and duration of exercise, you may also be able to slowly decrease your insulin dosages.

What Is Meaningful Exercise?

Using exercise to lose fat, get in shape, and truly prevent diabetes requires regular, meaningful, long-duration exercise. In addition, diet is very important: how much you *don't* eat is far more important than how much you *do* move. The 20–30 minutes of exercise 3 times per week so often recommended to maintain marginal cardiovascular fitness is *not* enough to significantly affect body weight. In order to lose weight with aerobic exercise, it takes at least 1 hour per day of tough, continuous exercise, 6 or 7 days per week. Light walking, jogging, and aerobic dance bring you only to a state of normalcy. The reason for this is quite simple: You have the physiology of a Stone Age hunter-gatherer, so inactivity is abnormal for you and activity is normal. That is the fundamental reason why everyone feels so much better when they start a regular exercise program. Your body is designed to be active and mobile every day of your life, and you ignore nature at great peril. If your weight or your weakness has been preventing you from exercising, or even freely negotiating a flight of steps, you have been denying your body one of its most fundamental needs—mobility.

In one study, Japanese diabetics reversed their disease simply by walking 6 miles per day. We have to keep in mind that our normal glucose metabolism is adapted to a life of strenuous and lengthy bouts of exercise, which were mandatory to sustain life. Nobody in Paleolithic times could arbitrarily stop chasing game and sit down with a bowl of chips in front of the TV. Even when agriculture was adopted, it was hardscrabble subsistence farming, as is the case in many developing countries today. Subsistence farming is all-day manual labor and a far cry from modern agricultural production and supermarket shopping.

Meaningful exercise always recognizes that losing fat is the issue, not losing weight. You want to keep your muscles! Muscle is a precious commodity and, once lost, is rarely regained without tremendous effort. *Performing aerobic exercise (and dieting) without regard to muscle wasting is fruitless and self-defeating.* All forms of exercise, to a greater or lesser degree, either damage or burn muscle tissue for energy. In a meaningful exercise and diet program, we want to minimize loss of muscle and, if possible, increase muscle mass. We have already discussed the difference between being skinny and being lean. Very often, aerobic exercise fanatics, especially long-distance runners, lose large amounts of muscle and become skinny, *not* lean. What's more, a good deal of the weight loss benefit from aerobic exercise is really from the diversionary aspect—you don't eat while you exercise.

Muscles are active tissue and burn calories 24 hours per

day. The bigger, leaner, and more muscular you are, the higher your resting metabolism. This is the reason why a large male bodybuilder can burn more calories per hour sitting on the sofa than the average woman does running! While the overall calculation of the resting metabolic rate is very complex, a good rule of thumb is 10 calories per pound of lean body mass per day. Since most women do not have more than 120 pounds of lean body mass, they can't eat more than about 1,200 calories per day if they want to lose fat. It is not unusual, however, for a man to have 170–200 pounds of lean body mass, which means that 1,700 or 2,000 calories per day will not sustain him beyond lying at rest all day. Thus, the overall best way to lose fat is to follow the Modern Evolutionary Diet, starting with an exercise program that increases your muscle mass and strength. Alternate weightlifting with moderate aerobic exercise if you can, but if you have to choose only one, or limit exercise due to time or health constraints, a few hours a week spent lifting weights are far better than a few hours spent on aerobics in terms of body fat loss.

If you're still not convinced, consider this study at the University of Colorado. The study found that running elevates the metabolism and burns body fat (if you don't eat right away) for 1 hour after exercise, but weightlifting elevates the metabolism for 15 hours after exercise.

Weight training to increase muscle strength and mass is where you really do the grunt work to put your body back in fighting form. People of any age or state of health can lift weights! In fact, the latest research shows that weight training is the single most important thing that the elderly can do to prevent loss of balance, coordination, strength, and mobility. The gains seniors can make in these areas, as well as lowering blood pressure and glucose, are nothing short of extraordinary. Remember as well that every health club has trainers to help you, should you need them.

I've been a lifelong athlete, exercising an hour or more every day, and at times 3 to 6 hours per day. The most significant parts of my regimen are the three days I spend weight lifting. I use a very intense form of training in which weights are lifted and lowered very slowly, called Super Slow. At this intensity, my exercising is crunchingly anaerobic *and* aerobic at the same time, yet with little risk of injury. Acceleration is the major source of sports injury. If you have time for only one athletic endeavor, this is the one to do. You can do Super Slow one day per week and be in vastly better shape than a person who jogs every day.

Meaningful exercise always recognizes the difference between exercise and recreation. Exercise is performed at a high level of intensity, and exercise significantly and continually increases the strength and endurance of the exerciser. Recreation is fun and relaxation, and getting stronger and fitter is not its primary purpose. Ideally, we would like to have these two words be one and the same, so that the pursuit of meaningful exercise becomes your recreation. It is important that you choose the kind of exercise that suits you, or else you will not be willing to put in the effort it takes to really get in shape, lose fat, and reverse or prevent diabetes. No diet or supplement plan can reach its full effectiveness if you are overfat and sedentary.

Choose the exercise you like to do, and what you are able to do. Generally, the safest and most productive exercise regimen involves alternating weight lifting and aerobic exercise, such as running, bicycling, walking, or swimming. These improve blood circulation, body composition, and strength. Weight lifting is certainly recommended for those whose cardiovascular system is healthy. If you, for example, suffer from high blood pressure, you may need to be careful with both weight lifting and rigorous aerobic exercise. You may need to lose some weight before you can accomplish much heavy exercise. You may not be able to do *anything* but walk at first.

Keep in mind that we neither gain nor lose weight overnight — both take time, and your resting metabolism slows as you age. You have to make any effort you can to exercise daily. If you are dieting and food cravings hit, do some exercises for a few minutes and you will be amazed to find that the food cravings have greatly diminished. Exercise is also helpful for reducing cigarette cravings and eyestrain, headaches, or muscle pain caused by sitting at a desk too long. In fact, as soon as the craving hits to put something in your mouth, take whatever opportunity you can to exercise briefly, wherever you are. Don't, for example, use the fact that you are "busy at work" to give you an excuse for avoiding a quick 10 minutes of exercise. If you are trapped at home, take the kids around the block, clean out the basement, rearrange some heavy furniture, or put on some favorite music and dance a little.

Super Slow Training

Author Pasquale "Pat" Covelli has had Type I diabetes for 34 years. He has many complications, including retinopathy, nephropathy, and peripheral vascular disease. Pat has had a kidney transplant, and prior to that he was on kidney dialysis. He has also had two bypass operations in his legs and he has 8½ feet of scar tissue from various surgeries. He had an Achilles tendon removed and five toes amputated. Still, he's not giving up, and after weight training with the Super Slow method, he's really holding his own and even working on a new book.

"I started Super Slow training after I had my kidney transplant," Pat said. "I got Robert Francis, a master Super Slow instructor, weight trainer, and rehabilitation specialist, to train me at my home. It's the only system of exercise that makes sense for people like me with such compromised health. I also needed a form of exercise that could get me back in shape without further damaging my eyes or kidneys. I was extremely thin after my surgery—less than 120 pounds, and I had lost a lot of muscle. Now I weigh 149 pounds, having put on only muscle. I'm so much stronger, and I've had no further progression of my peripheral vascular disease. My two surgeries for this occurred before I started training."

He continued: "As if I wasn't in bad enough shape already, I also broke my hip while recovering from the kidney transplant. The hospital rehabilitation staff gave up on me, but Bob did not! I was in a wheelchair for a year, and couldn't even get up the stairs—I lived on one floor of the house. Now I'm completely mobile and holding my complications at bay." Pat experienced somewhat better glucose control and a huge increase in stamina as a result of training, but didn't notice any drastic lowering of his insulin requirements. This isn't unexpected, since Pat has Type I diabetes and is underweight, not overweight. However, it's important to realize that the extra 30 pounds of muscle he's added have not increased his insulin requirements, whereas 30 pounds of fat would certainly be unhealthy and would raise insulin requirements.

More on Super Slow

Dennis Beckman, a master Super Slow instructor, trains clients one-on-one in slow, controlled, heavy lifting. Super Slow and similar types of training involve doing a single set, usually 10 seconds positive motion (lifting the weight up) and 10 seconds negative (lowering the weight down). The training pushes muscles beyond failure, which results in large strength and lean body mass gains for little investment in time. The technique is very safe, even for those who are elderly or in poor physical condition.

Washington attorney John Reilly is 70 years old and a Type II diabetic whose disease has progressed so far that he needs to take insulin. He admits to being overweight and not making much of an effort to exercise. He came to Dennis for Super Slow training. Dennis remarked, "John responded to training very quickly, and he got much stronger, despite his age and diabetes. I only wish he'd come more regularly!" Dennis has seen other individuals with impaired glucose tolerance or diabetes improve noticeably, as they increase their strength and lean body mass and decrease body fat.

John also noticed that he's stronger and his blood sugar is lower than it's ever been. He said, "It's under control, not scary, you know—it runs from 100 to 120 mg/dl, which isn't bad at all. I also started taking a new medication about the same time I started weight training, so I'm not sure which factor was the most important, but between the two things, I've substantially cut down on insulin. I've also noticed that eating a lot of fat makes my blood sugar go up, so I'm more careful about that."

Recently John stopped training for 4–5 months, and he noticed that the only complication he has—some neuropathy—came back during the time he quit. The return of this complication is likely to be due to poorer blood sugar control, so he's getting ready to resume his workouts.

Moderate Exercise Does *Not* Require More Carbohydrates!

Most people overestimate how many calories they burn while exercising, and very often don't lose weight because they spend a lot of time rewarding themselves with sugary foods, sports drinks, or favorite meals. The number of calories consumed in the bottle of Gatorade that many people swill after working out is more than they have burned during the exercise! What's worse is that the huge pure carbohydrate dose in the Gatorade may satisfy immediate hunger pangs, but the pangs come back in a hour or so with a vengeance. Unlike your resting metabolism, calories burned during exercise correlate with your total weight. If you are heavy or obese, your muscles are doing weight lifting all the time to haul around your storage fat! While diligent aerobic exercise can aid weight loss, it cannot work without a concerted effort at dieting, unless you are doing something really tough, such as training for competition. In fact, high-carbohydrate sport drinks and meal replacements do have legitimate uses for elite competition athletes. They train hours daily and must always attempt to better their last performance while not suffering injury. Unfortunately, these high-carbohydrate drinks and foods are marketed to the average person, who has little need or use for them.

People who start a regular exercise program are led to believe that they need more carbohydrates. Unless you are a pro athlete or lumberjack, this is not the case at all! Moderate exercise most days of the week for normal individuals trying to keep fit requires about 20–50 extra grams of protein (80–200 calories) and 5–15 grams of polyunsaturated fatty acids (45–135 calories) per day. A single doughnut might have this many calories, but not the nutrients. If you eat the doughnut, you *still* require the protein and the polyunsaturated fatty acids calories to function optimally. Again, the doughnut is so nutrient poor, it does not contain enough vitamins and minerals to metabolize the calories. Your body must borrow them from somewhere else. A successful exercise program for you may well require extra essential nutrients, but does not require extra calories, especially in the form of carbohydrates.

Supplements to Help Your Breathing and Circulation

What do you do if your mind wants to exercise, but your body will not cooperate? If you have been overweight, diabetic, smoking, or sedentary for some time, you may have damaged or atrophied muscles, lungs, heart, and blood circulation. If you have tried to exercise and have no wind, or your legs feel so heavy or achy that they can't respond, do not despair. First off, you must be patient and give yourself time to heal and lose fat. But although patience is a virtue, there are specific supplements you can take to speed your physiological recovery and jump-start your exercise program. You don't need to follow this program forever—only until you feel you are back in fighting form. However, if these are chronic problems for you, you might need to keep taking a few of these supplements indefinitely. In any case, all the supplements are safe, clinically tested for these conditions, and not contraindicated for medications.

You can test your ability to exercise with the WALK/RUN TALK method. If you can walk or run while talking to a partner, your heart rate is in a safe range. If you don't have a partner, sing or recite aloud. If you are panting, gasping for breath, or unable to carry on a normal conversation, you need to slow down your pace and then work daily at a slower pace, building up strength gradually. Keep using the WALK/RUN TALK check to see how you are doing.

To Improve Respiratory Function

These suggestions are for those with coughing, wheezing, shortness of breath, chronic bronchitis, or mild asthma or chronic obstructive pulmonary disease (COPD).

If you have severe asthma or COPD that must be controlled with medications, other natural approaches can help you more than those listed here. However, they are beyond the scope of this book. Consult a physician who is knowledgeable in the nutritional and pharmaceutical management of these conditions, and check the Resources section. In general, very safe mild bronchodilation can be accomplished with the suggestions below, but substitute 1 capsule of Coleus forskohlii herb 3 times per day for the emblica/triphala. Use a product standardized for 1 mg of forskohlii. *Make sure you also use RespirActin and vitamin C!* You can use or omit fritillary, if you wish.

- Antioxidants are a must. Use a broad-spectrum antioxidant, and also take 1,000 mg vitamin C with bioflavonoids 3 times per day.

- Multivitamin/multimineral with at least 30 mg of each B in the B complex.
- Additional 400 mg magnesium per day.
- RespirActin: 2 ounces twice per day.
- N-acetyl-cysteine: 500 mg 3 times per day. If your physician can provide you with an inhaler, use it.
- Curcumin: 1 capsule 3 times per day.
- Emblica herb, fritillary herb, or Triphala (an Ayurvedic herbal blend): 1 capsule/tablet of any one 3 times per day. You can also alternate these, or look for blends of these herbs.
- Strongly recommended: Regular use of bee pollen and, even better, royal jelly and propolis combination supplementation.
- Optional: Grape seed or pine bark extract.

To Improve Peripheral Circulation

Ailments of the peripheral circulation include peripheral vascular disease, varicose veins, phlebitis, hemorrhoids, swollen ankles (edema), and heavy or weak legs.

- Antioxidants are a must. Use a broad-spectrum antioxidant supplement. Also take vitamin E at 600–800 IU for 6–10 weeks, then drop back to 400 IU.
- Multivitamin/multimineral with at least 30 mg of each B in the B complex.
- Additional 400 mg magnesium per day.
- Tibetan Formula No. 28: 1 tablet 3 times per day. This is an ancient Tibetan blend of herbs designed specifically for conditions with impaired circulation, such as intermittent claudication.
- Garlic: 2 capsules or tablets 2 or 3 times per day.
- Centella Asiatica and/or bilberry: 1 capsule 3 times per day. You can use one or the other, both, alternate both, or look for a combination product. Use a product that contains standardized extract in a whole herb base.

- L-carnitine: 1,000 mg three times per day on an empty stomach.
- Strongly recommended: Regular use of bee pollen and, even better, royal jelly and propolis combination supplementation.
- Optional: Grape seed or pine bark extract.

For severe, recurrent phlebitis or bad varicose veins, add 1 capsule each of rutin and horse chestnut (also a standardized product) 3 times per day. Also add bromelain enzyme at 200 mg 3 times per day, or 400–500 mg twice per day on an empty stomach. You can also look for blends with these herbs.

For recurrent hemorrhoids, add 1 capsule of butcher's broom herb 3 times per day. If this is your only problem, you can skip the extra vitamin E, L-carnitine, Tibetan Formula No. 28, and garlic, if you wish.

For Persistent Fatigue

If you are just too tired to get started or want to quit as soon as you have started, here are a few suggestions. The three herbs are best if used all together and may take a few weeks to kick in.

- Start on the Modern Evolutionary Diet and supplement plan first for 2–6 weeks. Antioxidants, green power foods, and a high-potency multivitamin are a must.
- Additional 400 mg magnesium per day.
- Korean ginseng herb: 1 capsule or tablet 3 times per day.
- Schizandra: 1 capsule or tablet 3 times per day.
- Jade Chinese Stamina blend: 2 or 3 tablets 30 minutes before exercising.
- Optional: Royal jelly, 1 capsule 3 times per day, and RespirActin, 1 ounce twice per day.

4

Chromium and Other Trace Nutrients That Influence Glucose Metabolism and Diabetes

Vitamins and trace elements can directly influence our glucose metabolism. If these particular nutrients are lacking in the diet, we may be more susceptible to diabetes, or the nutrient deficiency may be a *direct cause* of Type II diabetes. In the cases of chromium and B complex vitamins, deficiencies definitely can cause diabetes. The nutrients discussed in this chapter are important for diabetes prevention and reversal.

Chromium

Chromium is an essential trace element required for normal insulin functioning. Chromium deficiency can *directly cause* Type II diabetes, and causes the symptoms of high fasting blood sugar, poor glucose tolerance, and decreased binding of insulin to insulin receptors. The number of insulin receptors on our cells can also decrease, further increasing the risk for abnormally high levels of both blood sugar and insulin. While it's a dangerous situation to have high blood sugar, it's also dangerous to have chronically high levels of insulin circulating in the blood. This means not only that the insulin isn't being used effectively, but it's also an independent risk factor for heart disease, high blood pressure, obesity, and chronic inflammatory conditions. Chronically high or unbalanced levels of any hormone are not beneficial for humans.

Chromium deficiency can also lower blood plasma HDL ("good") cholesterol, while raising total plasma cholesterol, LDL ("bad") cholesterol, and triglycerides (triacylglycerols). Since anyone with Types I or II diabetes is at increased risk for cardiovascular disease, improving cholesterol and triglyceride profiles by supplementing chromium may provide additional benefits.

Typical North American and European diets require more chromium than they provide, which leads to long-term depletion of body chromium reserves. Much research has estimated that 90 percent of the U.S. population does not obtain the Estimated Safe and Adequate Daily Dietary Intake (ESADDI) of 50 to 200 micrograms (mcg) per day of chromium. Similar research results have been observed in Canada, the United Kingdom, and Finland.

It's very important to realize that *a diet high in refined grains and sugars exacerbates chromium depletion.* First, these foods contain low amounts of chromium, yet chromium is necessary to metabolize them. Second, a high consumption of sugars and refined carbohydrates increases chromium excretion in the urine by 10–300 percent.

Sometimes a person can "pass" a glucose tolerance test when the pancreas produces abnormally high amounts of insulin to metabolize the glucose. This poses a problem for optimum chromium nutrition, because high levels of insulin circulating in the blood also increase the amount of chromium excreted in the urine, but at the same time *increase* the body's requirements for chromium. This happens because chromium is a cofactor for insulin, and so the higher the amounts of insulin, the more chromium is required. Without chromium supplementation or dietary changes, over time insulin levels get progressively higher and glucose tolerance gets progressively worse, eventually resulting in diabetes.

Exercise activates insulin receptors in the muscle cells.

Glucose uptake by the muscle cells is greatly enhanced compared to resting conditions. This glucose uptake requires concomitant action by chromium, but it does not appear that chromium is efficiently recycled by the body. Unfortunately, chromium excretion in the urine increases significantly following exercise. This means that athletes may have increased requirements for chromium. It also means that if you exercise regularly to help control diabetes, it is essential that you supplement chromium.

Chromium Availability in the Diet

Brewer's yeast, beer, whole grains, cheese, liver, and meat can be good dietary sources of chromium; however, the chromium contents of foods vary widely. Much of the chromium measured in foods may actually be unabsorbable, because it originates from metal contamination from stainless steel food-processing equipment. Refining of grains and sugars and processing of foods remove most of the absorbable chromium.

Chromium absorption *decreases* with increasing dietary intake at levels below 40 mcg. Above 40 mcg, absorption appears to remain constant at a very low percentage of intake. This means, in effect, that our bodies work more to protect us from high levels of chromium and similar trace elements than they do to combat diabetes. Apparently, our bodies cannot make much of an adjustment to today's high-calorie, high-carbohydrate, refined, nutrient-poor diets and increase chromium absorption appropriately.

Unlike most of the trace elements that are essential for mammals, chromium has not been shown to be essential for plants, and so plants don't make an effort to concentrate it. Chromium levels depend simply on how and where various plants are grown. Accordingly, fruits, vegetables, grains, and legumes intrinsically contain varying amounts of chromium. Soils with abundant chromium must of necessity develop from underlying rocks rich in chromium, which are rare in the earth's crust.

How to Supplement Chromium

The biologically active form of chromium may be a nicotinic acid-amino acid complex. The amino acids in this complex contain at least glycine, cysteine, and glutamic acid. This complex was first isolated from extracts of brewer's yeast and was named the glucose tolerance factor (GTF). It was observed that rats became diabetic when the GTF yeast was not in their diets, but regained normal glucose tolerance when it was returned. It is known that chromium is much less effective if nicotinic acid (vitamin B_3) is deficient, and that the converse is true also—nicotinic acid alone cannot prevent diabetes if chromium is deficient.

The isolation of GTF led to the notion that "GTF chromium" is the preferred supplemental form. In fact, the structure of yeast-derived GTF is still unknown, but it *is* known that the chromium does not need to be provided in the exact GTF form to be effective. This is like assuming that only ground-up human bone can be ingested as a source of calcium for growing our bones. The body takes in nutrients in a variety of forms, and then manufactures complexes and structures within our bodies to do tasks as required. So far, all the GTF complex synthetic supplements that I have examined are nothing but messy mixtures of amino acids, nicotinic acid, water, and chromium salts. They may or may not be effective chromium supplements, depending on the manufacturer. The major problems are the lack of stability and consistency in the raw material.

The chromium supplement shown to be both the most effective and best absorbed is chromium picolinate, and this is the one I recommend. A recent double-blind placebo-controlled study on three groups of 60 Chinese diabetes patients found that 500 mcg of chromium picolinate given twice per day for 4 months was greatly superior to a placebo in lowering fasting and post-meal blood glucose and nearly normalizing glycated hemoglobin (a test used to measure the extent of diabetes). Total cholesterol and insulin levels also dropped. A third group given 100 mcg twice per day showed lesser but significant improvements in glycated hemoglobin and insulin levels, but not blood glucose levels.

Since nicotinic acid is a vitamin, it was considered that it would be good (and marketable) to chelate chromium with nicotinic acid. However, the chemical structure of nicotinic acid does not lend itself to chemical bonding with chromium. In my own research, I have found that in the "chromium polynicotinate" compound chromium is bonded to water and/or hydroxide (OH), not nicotinic acid. Chromium picolinate has been also shown to be better absorbed by rats than chromium polynicotinate in side-by-side comparison. I would note, also, that no chromium compound has ever been shown to be toxic at normal doses or even doses thousands of times greater than normal.

Some unscrupulous marketing has been associated with chromium nicotinate, polynicotinate, and so-called GTF chromium supplements. Nicotinic acid (vitamin B_3) in doses of 200–2,000 mg can help lower cholesterol, blood sugar, and possibly reduce the risk of heart attacks, and so chromium-nicotinic acid supplements have been promoted for these conditions. This is very misleading, because the amount of nicotinic acid in a 200 mcg chromium supplement is less than 1 mg, which is insignificant with respect to the 200–2,000 mg effective dosage range, and even with respect to the RDA level of 14–19 mg. Since both chromium and vitamin B_3 are important nutrients, the best nutritional forms of each should be supplemented, but not necessarily in the same chemical compound.

This example sets a good rule to apply to all nutritional supplements. Although combining everything in a few pills per day is convenient and may make for exciting marketing, it is often impossible to set up a good program in that manner. The dosages, as well as the form of the supplement, are going to be severely compromised. Treat your body with respect, and give it what it needs to heal and thrive!

Appropriate dietary choices and chromium supplementation of 200–400 mcg per day may help prevent Type II diabetes, but may not be sufficient to reverse existing diabetes. To reverse existing diabetes, chromium picolinate is recommended at 1,000–1,200 mcg per day, in two to four divided doses. If you are taking any medication to control your blood sugar, start with 200 mcg per day for a week and monitor your glucose closely. Increase the dosage by 200 mcg per week until you reach 1,000 mcg and then have medication adjusted accordingly.

For Type I diabetes, use the same approach. Add chromium in 100–200 mcg increments per week. Monitor glucose closely, because you should experience a decrease in your insulin requirements. If you have trouble adjusting the insulin dose you take just before going to bed, do not take chromium supplements within 3 hours of retiring. Work up to the level of chromium that allows you to consistently reduce your daytime insulin, and stabilize your requirements. Then work on the night dosage.

Chromium and Diabetes

Richard A. Anderson, Ph.D., is a nutritional biochemist at the Nutrient Requirements and Functions Laboratory of the USDA Beltsville Human Nutrition Research Center in Maryland. He has been working on the nutritional role of chromium in diabetes and cardiovascular diseases for more than 20 years. Considered the most prominent expert in this field, he says that the evidence for the beneficial effects of chromium on diabetes gets stronger each year.

I asked him to explain how Type I and Type II diabetics differ in their requirements and usage of chromium. "Chromium functions by improving the efficiency of insulin," Dr. Anderson said. "It does not replace insulin. In Type I diabetes, insulin is not produced by the body and therefore chromium has minimal effects. Some studies, however, have demonstrated that even in Type I diabetes chromium decreases insulin requirements. In Type II diabetes, the problem in more than 75 percent of the cases is too much insulin, yet the insulin is not effective. Chromium improves the effectiveness of the insulin, leading to lower levels of circulating blood glucose and also lower circulating insulin. Insulin concentration decreases due to the increased efficiency, and therefore less insulin is required."

I asked him whether he saw the use of chromium as a pharmaceutical supplement for diabetes within 5 years. "Presently supplemental chromium is being taken by a large segment of the population with Type II diabetes," Dr. Anderson replied. "This is one reason why we did our most recent chromium supplementation study in China, since most of the subjects recruited in the United States were either taking individual chromium supplements or other supplements that also contained chromium. The number of people with diabetes also taking supplemental chromium will increase dramatically as the medical community becomes more aware of the overwhelming evidence documenting a role of chromium in the prevention, alleviation, and treatment of diabetes. Chromium is *not* a drug used in the treatment of diabetes, but a nutrient that functions in the normal control of glucose, insulin, blood lipids, and related risk factors associated with diabetes and cardiovascular diseases."

Dr. Anderson and I have been working together on chromium and cinnamon for potential diabetic treatments for the past four years, but I defer to him when we need to discuss mechanisms of action. Here's his best guess as to the mechanism of action of chromium, and how it's apparently similar to the action of the effective molecule from cinnamon: "Chromium functions at a number of places in the mechanism of action of insulin," Dr. Anderson said. "Chromium increases insulin binding to cells by increasing the number of insulin receptors on the cells. In order for insulin to function in the control of glucose, it must bind to these receptors. Chromium also regulates enzymes at the insulin receptor level. It regulates these enzymes to increase the number of phosphate groups bound to specific insulin receptor proteins. The more bound phosphate groups, the more sensitive cells are to insulin, leading to increased insulin efficiency. Chromium and cinnamon are likely to function by similar mechanisms, since both appear to regulate glucose through their interaction with insulin."

B Vitamins

All B vitamins are fundamental to our energy metabolism. A multivitamin with at least 30 mg of each B in the B complex, 30 mcg of vitamin B_{12}, and 400 mcg of folic acid is an essential part of the basic supplement plan and cannot be omitted. Your multivitamin should also contain biotin, choline, inositol, and PABA at around the same levels of the B complex (but microgram levels for biotin, as for vitamin B_{12}). If your multivitamin has 50–100 mg of each B in the B complex and related B vitamins, this is likely to be sufficient. If not, there are several B vitamins that are especially important for diabetics, and you may want to piggy-back an extra 30–60 mg per day onto your basic plan.

Vitamin B_3

Vitamin B_3 (the common forms are niacin, nicotinic acid, and nicotinamide) is essential for glucose metabolism. One of the symptoms of gross B_3 deficiencies is a diabetic-like condition. Chromium is not effective if nicotinic acid is deficient, and vice versa. B_3 has also been used at 500–2,000 mg per day levels to slow the progression of Type I diabetes and fairly severe Type II diabetes with complications, but this should be done only under the advice and care of a professional!

Natural Treatments

Kathleen Head, N.D., an expert in natural treatments for Type I diabetes, was in private practice in San Diego for 11 years before joining Thorne Research in Sandpoint, Idaho. She finds that Type I diabetes patients don't always respond to treatments such as *Gymnema sylvestre*, chromium, and vanadium the way Type II diabetes patients do. "You have to be careful when you start on these treatments and monitor Type I diabetes patients closely," she said. "I think some of the natural treatments may compete with injected insulin instead of helping it." However, she finds that natural treatments for preventing and treating diabetic complications, especially antioxidants and herbs, are effective for all diabetics. Dr. Head has designed a diabetic supplement for Thorne which contains *Gymnema sylvestre*, alpha lipoic acid, quercetin, bilberry, chromium, and vanadium. "I chose the quercetin because it's an aldose reductase inhibitor and thus can help diabetic retinopathy and cataracts," she said. "Bilberry is also beneficial to the eyes and is a collagen stabilizer."

Dr. Head commented about diabetic patients in general: "It's hard to get patients to test their blood sugar regularly on their own. Regular testing is really important because it lets us know how the treatments are working, and whether we need to make adjustments to the program. It's also just good practice for staying healthy and minimizing complications."

Vitamin B$_6$

Vitamin B$_6$ deficiency is clearly related to symptoms of diabetes. The active form of vitamin B$_6$, known as pyridoxal phosphate, is absolutely required for the proper metabolism of carbohydrates. B$_6$ deficiency can cause high blood sugar, abnormal glucose tolerance, reduced insulin secretion, degeneration of the beta cells of the pancreas that produce insulin, and reduced insulin sensitivity. Both males and females wishing to prevent or reverse Type II diabetes should have a multivitamin with at least 30 mg B_6 as part of their basic supplement plan, but B_6 is of special concern for women. Vitamin B_6 is one of the vitamins that is required for regulating the menstrual cycle, and for pregnancy and nursing.

Women taking birth control pills both need and excrete more B_6, and can sometimes have symptoms including leg muscle cramps, carpal tunnel syndrome, and a degeneration of their blood sugar control. Lack of B_6 is also implicated in premenstrual syndrome (PMS). In both of these cases, supplementing at least 30 and more typically 50–100 mg B_6 has been shown to be helpful. The symptoms of leg muscle cramps, carpal tunnel syndrome, irritability, or fluid retention, as well as active diabetes, often occur later in the term of a pregnancy. Women who are not normally diabetic sometimes become diabetic during pregnancy, a condition known as gestational diabetes.

Gestational diabetes is much more similar to Type II than Type I diabetes, and the incidence of gestational diabetes basically follows the same ethnic trends that are observed for Type II diabetes. Gestational diabetes is very prevalent among Hispanic and Native American groups, and is more common in American blacks and Asians than Caucasians. It is also more prevalent in older mothers. My basic recommendations for Type II diabetes prevention and treatment apply to gestational diabetes: Exercise, don't gain too much weight, supplement basic vitamins and trace elements, take extra chromium, follow the Modern Evolutionary Diet for weight maintenance, and increase dietary protein while decreasing carbohydrates. In addition, I would specifically emphasize supplementing 50–100 mg vitamin B_6, 800 mcg chromium picolinate, and 400-600 mg magnesium per day for pregnant women at risk for gestational diabetes.

Vitamin D

These days vitamin D is a sleeper nutrient that is hardly ever on anyone's list. However, as we move into a new era in which the population of elderly persons is as large as or larger than the population of children, we will have to reconsider this situation. Vitamin D differs from all other essential nutrients in that humans are capable of manufacturing all they need. The precusor molecule for vitamin D is 7-dehydrocholesterol, and converting it to vitamin D takes only 20–30 minutes of exposure to the sun about half the days of the week. It was learned early in the century that rickets in children could be cured by exposing them to ultraviolet light. Rickets became common around the time of the industrial revolution, when children began to spend long hours indoors in schools, inner-city homes, and factories. The same type of situation is happening now with elderly Americans. They are living years or even decades in retirement and nursing homes, with little if any regular outdoor activity. Even those who retire to sunny places such as Florida and Arizona find themselves virtual slaves to the comfort of air conditioning and apply SPF 30 sunscreen for up to 9 months of the year. It is estimated that 30–50 percent of the elderly are vitamin D deficient!

This lack of vitamin D is a serious concern for immune function and bone and muscle strength in the elderly. Lack of vitamin D has also been linked to glucose intolerance in the elderly, and quite possibly coronary artery disease, heart attack, and chronic respiratory infections. With respect to glucose intolerance, 14 elderly Dutch men (ages 70–88) had their vitamin D levels tested. Thirty-nine percent were vitamin D depleted. They were given a 1 hour glucose tolerance test, and those with lower blood levels of vitamin D had greater areas under the glucose tolerance curve. Levels of insulin were also higher during the test in those with lower vitamin D. This means that, all other factors being equal, the men's performance on the glucose tolerance test was worse if they had low levels of vitamin D. Although this type of test identifies a potential risk factor for diabetes, it does not demonstrate that a lack of vitamin D directly *causes* Type II diabetes. However, I expect that such research is forthcoming, and we can't neglect the fact that 39 percent of the men in the study were clinically deficient in vitamin D. This alone is cause for concern.

With respect to coronary artery disease and heart attacks, the evidence is a little more hypothetical and controversial, but very intriguing. And it helps explain my vitamin D recommendation for prevention and reversal of diabetes: Get outside as much as possible. Stick only to the 400 IU of vitamin D in your multivitamin and whatever you get in your food, and rely on the vitamin D your body makes from sunlight exposure. Let's look at why I've changed my approach here and asked you not to expect supplements to help you this time.

Vitamin D is needed to absorb calcium. After it was understood that a lack of either calcium or vitamin D caused rickets, dairy products and some other foods were supplemented with vitamin D, and cod liver oil became popular. However, there is little evidence that the effectiveness of supplemental vitamin D is anywhere close to naturally synthesized vitamin D. The concentration of vitamin D in our blood plasma increases in the summer and decreases in the winter. This pattern is totally independent of the supply of vitamin D in the diet, and reflects only the longer hours of daylight and greater opportunity for outdoor activities that summer provides. People who overwinter in Antarctica or spend long periods of time in submarines or orbiting spacecraft have strong decreases in their vitamin D levels, despite the fact that food supplemented with vitamin D is provided. Large oral doses of vitamin D result in toxic levels of vitamin D in the blood, whereas large doses of sunlight do not. The body closely regulates the synthesis of vitamin D in the skin, and its transport and uptake by the liver. Evidently this does not occur when vitamin D is taken as a supplement, and in fact D is one of the vitamins for which RDA levels are rarely exceeded. Unlike vitamin C, beta-carotene, and the B complex, supplemental vitamin D beyond what is necessary to prevent gross deficiency is not generally beneficial.

Northwest England, Scotland, Finland, and northern Sweden have very high incidences of coronary heart disease (blocked coronary arteries), often resulting in fatal heart attacks. Edinburgh and the surrounding areas of Scotland, in particular, have been the world leaders in heart attack fatalities for some time. This has been blamed on smoking, drinking, and the diet of the Scottish people. Certainly the Scots could improve their diet, but blaming their lifestyle alone doesn't hold up under scrutiny. People in France and Italy smoke, drink, and eat rich food too, but don't have anywhere near the incidence of coronary heart disease. This is known as the "French Paradox" and is particularly true of people who live in the south of France and in Sicily.

Consumption of red wine and more fruits, vegetables, fish, olive oil, and less fast food have been identified as plausible protective agents in the French diet. But equally or more powerful may be the protective effect of sunlight exposure.

Dr. David Grimes of Blackburn, England, hypothesized that the damage that initiates the blockage of arteries is the result of infection from the same type of bacteria that cause upper respiratory infections. Vitamin D confers resistance to these infections. Hence those living in sunny climates are less likely to have blocked coronary arteries, and less likely to have this condition progress to fatal heart disease. Grimes noted also that the molecule squalene is a common biochemical link between cholesterol and vitamin D (which is closely related to the cholesterol molecule). In the presence of sunlight, more squalene is converted into vitamin D, but in the absence of sunlight, more squalene is converted to cholesterol. So high cholesterol is a *marker* for an increased risk of coronary heart disease, because it marks a sunlight-deficient, vitamin D–deficient individual whose immune system is weakened. This explains why high cholesterol is identified as a risk factor for heart disease, but has never been shown to directly *cause* a heart attack. In fact, the relationship between dietary cholesterol intake and blood cholesterol levels is not very consistent, and simply lowering dietary cholesterol does little to help prevent heart attacks.

Zinc

Zinc levels tend to be lower than optimal in diabetics. In some cases, supplemental zinc has improved performance on glucose tolerance tests, but there is no consensus as to whether zinc supplementation makes significant improvements in blood sugar control in diabetics who are not grossly zinc deficient. It is generally agreed that moderate, but not excessive, zinc supplementation improves the overall metabolism of diabetics with very little cost or risk.

Zinc is involved in thousands of bodily functions. Our skin, hair, nails, bones, liver, mental acuity, senses, fat metabolism, circulatory, reproductive, and immune systems require zinc, and break down rapidly when it's lacking. All new tissue growth, eyesight, taste and smell, athletic performance, and dental health need zinc. Lack of zinc is a major factor in impotence, prostate problems, and infertility. Zinc is considered an antioxidant mineral, because it's a part of many enzymes that our bodies use to neutralize toxic substances.

Diets rich in animal protein usually supply enough zinc. The Modern Evolutionary Diet is designed to provide plenty of absorbable zinc, magnesium, and other trace elements. One drawback to high-fiber, low-protein, or vegetarian diets is potential zinc deficiency. Like iron, zinc is mainly associated with the protein content of foods.

Zinc from animal proteins is more bioavailable than from other sources. Oysters are among its richest sources. Lean red meat has twice as much zinc as does white meat such as poultry, but in general, meat and fish are the major sources of zinc in the diet. Dairy products, grains, and legumes provide much less. Fiber and two classes of phytochemicals, called phytates and oxalates, strongly interfere with zinc absorption. Phytates are found mostly in whole grains and legumes. Oxalates are found in grains, legumes, and some fruits and vegetables, such as rhubarb and spinach. Zinc can be absorbed at 30–50 percent efficiency from animal protein foods, but the zinc contained in whole grains and beans is absorbed at only 10–15 percent efficiency. The situation is similar with the absorption of iron. Zinc and iron deficiencies, for example, are common in developing countries where people exist on grains and beans, with very little animal protein. In contrast, typical hunter-gatherer diets provide no evidence for zinc deficiencies. The Modern Evolutionary Diet is designed to provide absorbable zinc in the diet every day.

If your multivitamin choice has 25–35 mg of zinc in the total daily dose, this is likely to be sufficient. If the levels are lower, take a 20–30 mg zinc supplement every other day. For certain health conditions, zinc supplementation at 50–100 mg per day is used, but this should be under the advice of a professional, and there is usually a drop-down to a lower maintenance dosage after a few weeks or months. These higher levels of zinc are not recommended for diabetics. Zinc picolinate, gluconate, aspartate, monomethione, and other amino acid chelated products are good choices for zinc supplements. Avoid zinc oxide and especially zinc sulfate, which can cause nausea for a short time after you take it.

Magnesium

Magnesium is consistently depleted in diabetics, especially those with Type I. Apparently, diabetes results in both higher magnesium requirements and excretion rates. Magnesium is a co-factor for glucose transport and helps regulate energy production. It functions in the production and release of insulin, and is required by cells for maintaining insulin sensitivity and increasing the number of insulin receptors. Magnesium is also needed for proper muscle and nerve function, including the heartbeat. This mineral is a major component of our bones and helps normalize blood pressure. In short, magnesium is critical to our health, and we can't live very long with a severe magnesium deficiency. If the deficiency is not classified as severe but rather suboptimal, we may remain alive but exist as the walking wounded.

Following the Modern Evolutionary Diet is a good way to naturally choose a diet high in magnesium. Hunter-gatherer diets were fairly high in magnesium. Vegetables (especially green vegetables, since magnesium is part of the chlorophyll molecule), fruits, meat, fish, shellfish, nuts, and dairy products are good food sources of magnesium. Significant magnesium is lost during food processing and cooking. Higher amounts of magnesium are found in raw and very lightly cooked fruits and vegetables (for example, steamed). When overcooked green vegetables take on a grayish cast, this means that the magnesium in the chlorophyll molecule has been replaced by hydrogen and is thus lost from the food. Whole grains have much greater amounts of magnesium per serving than refined grains, but, as is the case with zinc, phytates and fiber interfere with magnesium absorption.

A diet high in processed carbohydrate foods may not meet the daily magnesium requirements for a healthy person, and is definitely suboptimal for a person with diabetes.

If you don't eat fruits and vegetables, add both bee pollen and a green drink to your diet daily to help increase your magnesium intake. In addition to making dietary changes, 400–800 mg of supplemental magnesium should be taken per day. Unlike many other trace elements, magnesium is fairly well absorbed from a variety of inorganic (mineral salt as opposed to amino acid chelated) supplemental forms, so that magnesium oxide, hydroxide, and carbonate are fine to use. Magnesium citrate, aspartate, and lactate are better absorbed than oxides or carbonates, but you have to take more pills per day, since these sources are not as concentrated. Dolomite is not recommended as a magnesium or calcium supplement.

Note: If you have Type I diabetes or renal complications from diabetes or related kidney dysfunction, consult your physician before supplementing magnesium. Magnesium supplementation may not be beneficial for individuals whose excretion of mineral salts is impaired. In this case, it is best to stick to a diet sufficient in magnesium.

Antioxidants

Antioxidants include vitamin C, vitamin E, beta-carotene, selenium, zinc, and numerous botanical products such as grape seed, pine bark, green tea, and rosemary. Antioxidants are a must for preventing diabetic complications, and are part of the basic supplement plan for good health and fat loss. Antioxidants are synergistic and work best when all are supplemented together. Adequate supplemental levels of antioxidants may directly improve glucose tolerance and insulin sensitivity. Both vitamins C and E in excess of RDA levels have been supplemented in diabetics and diabetes-prone research animals. Both of these nutrients mainly help prevent cardiovascular and visual complications, but they also improve performance on glucose tolerance tests, and can reduce the insulin requirement for insulin-dependent diabetics.

In an animal study, 90 genetically diabetes-prone rats were fed either a high- or low-vitamin E diet for 90 days, or until they became diabetic. Only 5 of 45 animals on the high-vitamin E diet became diabetic, compared to 11 of 45 on the low-vitamin E diet. In only 3 months, low vitamin E apparently doubled the risk of developing diabetes in these rats. The typical Western diet, which is extremely low in vitamin E, is certainly not beneficial for preventing diabetes, and may in fact be detrimental. In a human study, very high doses of 900 mg (not IU) of vitamin E per day were given to 15 diabetes patients and 10 normal controls for 4 months. Glucose metabolism and tolerance were improved in both diabetic and normal subjects; however, the researchers did not advocate such high levels of supplementation without longer-term studies. This again makes an argument for taking vitamin E at 400–600 IU per day in the context of a total, balanced, antioxidant supplement. In one study of 241 humans, lower blood levels of vitamin C were correlated with higher levels of fasting blood sugar. In another study, patients visiting a clinic were given 500 mg of vitamin C twice per day for 10 days, and glucose tolerance improved in all patients.

The fruits and vegetables in the Modern Evolutionary Diet plan, coupled with the basic supplement plan's antioxidant and vitamin C suggestions, are sufficient levels of supplementation for those without diabetic complications. If you wish to add more vitamin C or botanical antioxidants, by all means go ahead. Just don't cheat on this part of the supplement plan, because you have nothing at all to gain and plenty to lose. If you now have diabetic complications, or if your diabetes is quite severe and you are at immediate risk for complications, see Chapter 13 for more aggressive and targeted antioxidant suggestions.

Note: If you have renal complications from diabetes or related kidney dysfunction, consult your physician before supplementing more than 1,000 mg of vitamin C three times per day (3,000 mg total).

L-carnitine

L-carnitine is useful for various diabetic complications, and there is also evidence that its supplementation can directly improve the impaired energy metabolism characteristic of diabetics. L-carnitine helps insulin work better, and helps control the hyperinsulinemia often symptomatic of Type II diabetes. L-carnitine also helps the body oxidize stored fat and improves overall lipid metabolism. L-carnitine can be made by the body, but apparently not everybody makes amounts that are optimal for health.

Diabetics appear to have a greater need for L-carnitine, yet excrete it at a greater rate than nondiabetic persons. L-carnitine is found naturally only in animal protein foods, especially in raw or rare meat. This is but another manifestation of how we are adapted to a hunter-gatherer diet, and how diabetes is caused by straying from that diet. Our modern diets, especially vegetarian diets, have little or no L-carnitine compared to hunter-gatherer diets.

L-carnitine is discussed in *The Carnitine Miracle* by Robert Crayhon. Recommended supplementation is 2–4 grams per day, and lower doses may not be effective. Since this is a naturally occurring amino acid, supplementation is very safe. The down side is that this is a very expensive supplement, and only a few suppliers have a high-quality product (see the Resources section).

What About Vanadium?

There is little doubt that vanadium can affect glucose metabolism, and in fairly large doses can lower blood sugar, but vanadium has never been demonstrated to be an essential trace element for humans. Even the often-quoted evidence for vanadium being essential for some other mammals is inconsistent, scanty, and unconvincing. Both humans and other mammals deprived of chromium become diabetic, and the diabetic symptoms can be reversed upon chromium supplementation. But nobody has shown that vanadium-deficient diets cause any harm to humans, and they certainly have not been shown to produce diabetic symptoms. In fact, there is no definition of a vanadium-deficient diet, because if this mineral is indeed essential, it is needed in such small quantities that enough is always present in a variety of diets. The effects of vanadium on blood sugar need to be considered pharmaceutical rather than nutritional.

Vanadium can help lower blood sugar if used properly, but it is considered pharmaceutical rather than nutritional for the following reasons: (1) Vanadium is not known to be an essential nutrient for maintaining health, (2) the toxicity of vanadium is quite high at relatively low doses, (3) the doses needed to significantly lower blood sugar are hundreds of times higher than the doses of chromium, a known nutritional factor, and (4) unlike chromium, vanadium has no effect on nondiabetic people.

Most research on vanadium has involved the form "vanadyl sulfate." However, supplementation of vanadyl sulfate is not advocated by any of the researchers who study it or by the U.S. Department of Agriculture. Recently, BMOV (bis-maltolato oxovanadium) and BGOV (bis-glycinato oxovanadate) have become available as alternatives to vanadyl sulfate in the United States and Canada. BMOV and BGOV are chelated forms of vanadium that may be more biologically active and absorbable. This means that less vanadium is needed to be effective for diabetes, and hence the potential for toxicity is lower.

The dosage of these chelated vanadium compounds and vanadyl sulfate for treating diabetes is 50–150 mg per day. Consult a professional before using vanadium on a long-term basis for controlling diabetes. Unlike chromium, vanadium *should not* be supplemented daily in order to prevent diabetes, because there is no evidence that it is an essential trace element or that it has benefits for people who are not diabetic.

5

Structural Fat Broadens Your Mind—Storage Fat Broadens Your Hips

Almost everyone is confused about the role of fats in their diet, and we get conflicting information from the media on a daily basis. This means that many of us don't know how much fat we should eat, or what types of fats are healthful. Fat is the most misunderstood macronutrient. Fat is not your enemy— it is as essential as protein. Dietary fats have *crucial* roles in the prevention and reversal of diabetes.

The three macronutrients in our diets are protein, carbo- hydrate, and fat. The word *macronutrient* refers to nutrients that we need to eat a lot of every day in order to have energy and materials to run and repair our bodies. The term *micronutrient* describes nutrients that we need only in trace amounts daily, such as vitamins. With regard to macronutri- ents, most people know that they need sufficient protein daily. But most people don't realize that although the body uses glucose as its fuel, it does not require (or even particu- larly desire) the ingestion of straight glucose. Glucose is a sugar, which is a carbohydrate, and we don't need very much carbohydrate per day to run our bodies properly. In fact, we can live our whole lives without eating *any* carbohydrates. However, we would all die without eating protein and fat.

What Are Dietary Fats?

All natural fats are mixtures of saturated (SFA), monoun-saturated (MUFA), and polyunsaturated fatty acids (PUFA). The exact compositions of natural fats can't be pinpointed, because they are dependent on factors such as growing conditions, plant or animal breeding, and processing. Therefore, we usually designate a fat as SFA, MUFA, or PUFA depending on what the *predominant* fatty acid type is. It is crucial to understand that no natural fats are intrinsically good or bad. Healthful fat nutrition requires nothing more than a balanced intake of these three types in minimally processed forms. The highly processed fats that line supermarket shelves are analogous to refined sugar. The nutrients needed to properly metabolize them and naturally prevent rapid spoilage (vitamins E and A, enzymes, antioxidant phytochemicals) have mostly been removed.

Polyunsaturated fatty acids have several double bonds in the carbon chain. Our bodies utilize PUFA in the *cis*-form. The term *cis* means that both hydrogens are on the same side of the double bond, like the relationship between your right foot and right hand, with your trunk as the double bond. In the *cis*-form the chains kink into a spiral structure. Thus they don't crystallize easily and remain liquid at refrigerator temperature. Some are also reactive, oxidizing and turning rancid relatively quickly, and should be stored in the refrigerator or frozen. However, this spirality, fluidity, and reactivity are absolutely essential to our metabolisms.

The group of PUFA (edible and nonedible, common and rare) contain a subgroup called essential fatty acids (EFA) — although there is no firm agreement on what fats are indeed essential. It is known that mammals cannot create PUFA from scratch, as they can SFA and MUFA. Therefore, PUFA is often equated with EFA, but this is a bit misleading as we shall see.

Monounsaturated fatty acids have a single double bond in the carbon chain. Liquid at room temperature, they partially crystallize and thicken upon refrigeration, for example, as olive oil does in the refrigerator overnight. Oleic acid, derived from its namesake salse, olives, is the most common and is present in virtually all vegetable oils; olive oil, peanut oil, and sesame oil are especially rich sources. Avocados and most nuts (i.e., pecans, Brazil nuts, almonds, walnuts, hazelnuts, and pistachios) have oleic acid. Oils high in monounsaturated fats keep reasonably well at cool room temperature for a few months, and even longer when refrigerated. They can be used as salad oil, in baking, and for light to medium heat sautéing.

Peanut oil can be used for stir-frying and deep frying, but most other vegetable oils cannot, unless they have been highly processed in order to stabilize them. Even so, it is impossible to completely prevent the breakdown of any oil at the 300–500 degrees F used in frying, so that all deep-fried foods are toxic to a greater or lesser degree and should be minimized in your diet.

Saturated fatty acids have no double bonds in the carbon chain and are solid at room temperature. Fats from land animals, found in meat, eggs, and dairy products, have a high percentage of saturated fat. Tropical oils such as cocoa, coconut, and palm oils also have a lot of saturated fat, as do macadamia nuts. Moderate amounts of saturated fat are healthful, and should never be denied to growing children. High amounts of saturated fat are not healthful, and tend to increase our risks for diabetes and cardiovascular disease.

The belief that tropical oils are unhealthful is discredited by the fact that millions in Southeast Asia have consumed these oils for millennia with a low incidence of cardiovascular disease. Human breast milk is approximately 45 percent saturated fat, including a large percentage of lauric acid, the same fatty acid that's prevalent in coconut oil. Lauric acid is critically important to prevent infections in infants. In addition, much of the saturated fat in tropical oils and dairy products consists of shorter carbon chains than meat fat and especially vegetable oils, and these shorter chains are more readily metabolized by our bodies. It is slightly easier for your body to burn coconut oil for energy than peanut or olive oil, for example; thus coconut oil used in prudent amounts is actually less likely to be stored on your hips and more likely to be burned for energy. This is not a license for overconsumption, just a call for moderation and a little common sense. Remember that no natural fats are intrinsically good or bad—it's the balance that matters most.

Clarified butter, ghee, and tropical oils can be stored at room temperature for 4–6 months or longer. Since saturated fats have no double bonds, they are much less chemically reactive. Saturated fats are the only fats that are universally recommended for frying or other high temperature cooking. Coconut oil and butter smoke at very low temperatures and cannot be used for frying, only low heat sautéing. Clarified butter, lard, and some palm oil preparations are suitable for higher temperature frying.

Artificial polyunsaturated fats include hydrogenated and high-temperature-processed vegetable oils. They all contain some percentage of *trans*-fatty acids. When oils are hydrogenated, the *cis* version switches to *trans* (like your right foot and left hand, with your trunk as the double bond) and the chain unkinks. The oil becomes solid (hence usable for baking) and very inert. Partially hydrogenated fats can sit for years on the shelf without spoiling—but what does this say about the nutritive value? Would you want to eat butter that had sat for a year on a shelf? Your cell walls and nervous tissue can't be constructed properly by eating mainly *trans*-polyunsaturated fats.

Trans-fats are marketed as polyunsaturated fats, but in terms of human health and metabolism they act more like saturated fats. *Trans*-fats were invented in a laboratory 90 years ago, and our cells haven't had enough evolution time to adapt to them. People consuming plenty of *trans*-fats poison themselves in the same way that a smoker or drug addict does. I recommend that *trans*-fats be minimized or avoided in your diet permanently. Margarine, shortening, the majority of commercial baked goods, candies, crackers, snack chips, and cocoa, pudding and dessert mixes all have hydrogenated fats. Read the labels!

Deep frying oil is filled with *trans* -fats also. Commercial frying oils are first partially hydrogenated to stabilize them. Then, every time they are heated up for frying, they react to form even more *trans* -fats from exposure to the high heat. Even worse, the scorching hot frying fats react strongly with oxygen in the atmosphere, forming literally hundreds of toxic compounds. For example, some Chinese women have a high rate of lung cancer, even though they rarely smoke. They stand over a wok every day, stir-frying in unrefined rapeseed (canola) oil and inhaling the toxic oil vapors. Canola and soybean oils can be toxic when used for deep or high temperature frying, and should be used mainly as salad or baking oils.

Glossary

EFA	Essential fatty acid
SFA	Saturated fatty acid
MUFA	Monounsaturated fatty acid
PUFA	Polyunsaturated fatty acid
LC-PUFA	Long-chain PUFA
n-3 PUFA	Omega-3 fatty acid
n-6 PUFA	Omega-6 fatty acid
LA	Linoleic acid
LNA	Alpha-linolenic acid
GLA	Gamma-linolenic acid
AA	Arachidonic acid
DHA	Docosahexaenoic acid
EPA	Eicosapentaenoic acid

Polyunsaturated Fatty Acids (PUFA)

By now we have all heard enough about what too much fat and cholesterol can do to our health. However, we are less aware of what the *lack* of certain fats can do to us. Specifically, the lack of omega-3 fatty acids (n-3 PUFA) in the diet is likely to be the single biggest nutritional deficiency in the United States. Like vitamins, PUFA are necessary to sustain human life and cannot be manufactured by our body. They can be obtained only through proper nutrition. PUFA are as critical to our health as protein, calcium, potassium, and other nutrients that we use in large quantities every day.

The body can manufacture both SFA and MUFA from other fats, protein, or carbohydrate. However, since the body cannot manufacture PUFA, SFA and MUFA cannot be used exclusively in any diet, unless you plan to live a short, miserable, disease-ridden life. If you are a strict vegetarian, for example, you must eat specific protein foods in order to get sufficient essential amino acids. Analogously, if you are not consuming certain fish, meats, and raw nuts in large quantities every day, you must choose supplemental oils to fulfill your PUFA requirements.

Junk food of all types, obesity, smoking, lack of antioxidants, lack of sunlight, and lack of balanced PUFA are major reasons why cardiovascular disease is our number one killer, and why diabetes continues to increase yearly. You can exercise yourself to exhaustion, cut all fat and cholesterol out of your diet, and eat nothing but beans, and you still may be at risk for diabetes and cardiovascular disease, if your diet lacks balanced intakes of unrefined, unprocessed PUFA.

Many of us would like to lose fat and everyone wants to be healthy. Low-fat and fat-free food products are very popular these days. There has been a tremendous effort to educate the public on the dangers of high-fat diets, and the media regularly provide low-fat cooking tips and recipes. Some low-fat diets have become so extreme, however, they cause people to increase their risk for chronic diseases while compromising their physical appearances. The reason is clear: These diets are extremely deficient in balanced PUFA.

It is possible to do yourself more harm than good with a very low-fat diet. Our skin and immune, digestive, cardiovascular, and neurological systems are dependent on PUFA.

Deficiencies in PUFA or metabolic abnormalities cause or contribute to chronic and acute diseases, including diabetes, cardiovascular disease, asthma, allergies, eczema, dermatitis, learning disabilities, multiple sclerosis, and schizophrenia. Humans need some fat, but what they don't need are excess calories. In this regard, there's a crucial distinction between structural fat and storage fat.

Structural Fat and Storage Fat

Structural fat is a major component of cell membranes, internal organs, and brain and nervous tissue. The myelin that sheathes our nerves is 79 percent fat! Structural fat always contains PUFA and thus cannot be constructed properly if PUFA are deficient. PUFA deficiencies during pregnancy and the first two years of a child's life, for example, can result in irreversible defects in the functioning of the child's nervous system and internal organs. Remember, though, that our ancestors existed on wild game, fish, shellfish, reptiles, and amphibians, which contain mainly structural fat as opposed to storage fat. Structural fat from wild game is typically balanced in PUFA, MUFA, and SFA, with very little intramuscular fat (marbling) and less than 7 percent total fat by weight.

Storage fat is largely saturated fat stored under our skin and on our abdomens, upper arms, hips, and thighs. Our ancestors purposely stored fat if they could, because they needed to carry around excess food for emergencies. We have kitchens and supermarkets to store food now, so we don't need much storage fat—but we continue to accumulate it! Our increasing excess in storage fat is mainly a consequence of straying from our evolutionary diet into processed foods loaded with sugar, refined grains, animal storage fat, and *trans*-fats. It is also a consequence of the low-cost availability of these foods 24 hours per day.

Despite the fact that we all require structural fat, its PUFA components have been systematically removed from the food supply in many Western countries. You simply cannot rely on commercial mass-produced foods to supply your balanced PUFA requirements. This is because natural PUFA are in the very perishable *cis* form, being easily destroyed by heating, processing, and moderate to high temperature cooking. They also turn rancid relatively rapidly, and so cannot be used in many products designed to sit on the grocery or cabinet shelf for months (or years!) unrefrigerated. Without adequate balanced PUFA, you can never look or feel your best, nor can you properly defend your body from disease, environmental toxins, or premature aging. Your physical and psychological abilities to make any profound changes in your health, diet, and lifestyle are severely hampered by PUFA as well as other nutrient deficiencies. This is not only because all nutrients are synergistic, but because part of your brain is made of PUFA.

LC-PUFA Derivatives

PUFA are conventionally defined in nutrition texts as linoleic acid and alpha-linolenic acid; both have 18 carbons in the fatty acid chain. Linoleic acid (LA) is the head of the n-6 PUFA family, and alpha-linolenic (LNA) is the head of the n-3 PUFA family. You can eat large amounts of LA and LNA, and in theory your body converts what it needs, with extra amounts being burned for energy or stored as body fat.

In practice, only small amounts of LA and LNA are converted by enzymes in your body into more biochemically active long-chain forms known as LC-PUFA derivatives. Diabetics have a strongly impaired ability to make these conversions. Diabetics and other people with poor LA and LNA conversion to LC-PUFA must eat or supplement direct sources of LC-PUFA to remain healthy.

N-6 PUFA

In the n-6 family, LA is in theory converted to the LC-PUFA derivatives gamma-linolenic acid (GLA) and arachidonic acid

(AA). In reality, only a few percent of dietary LA is actually converted. With respect to GLA, conversion may be so poor in the elderly, diabetics, and those with allergies and chronic skin and scalp disorders that GLA must be considered an EFA, and thus needs to be supplemented to maintain good health.

Complete conversion of LA to AA also occurs only to a very limited degree. Very little AA appears to be formed from LA in individuals consuming diets that contain animal foods. Some researchers have found that for normal Western diets, LA does not contribute to the formation of AA at all! When AA is consumed directly from animal fats, it is readily incorporated into our body's tissues. Furthermore, once AA is incorporated into cell membranes, it does not like to leave. Some people have written that you can "kick out" AA from your body's structural fat, and replace it with other fats. That's true, but it's not done so easily or so completely. Even worse is the popular misconception that you can marinate meat in vegetable oil and exchange AA in the meat with other fat. AA is put into structural fat and to a lesser extent storage fat by biochemical processes in the *living* organism that provided the meat, and short of digesting the meat, there is no way you can take AA out of the structure.

Individuals on vegan diets that have little or no AA but abundant LA have correspondingly low AA levels in their red blood cells. As exclusive carnivores, cats can't make this conversion at all, but omnivorous rats and mice are fairly good at making the conversion. Hence research on rodents may not be as applicable to humans in the case of dietary PUFA as it is in other cases. In humans, the conversion of LA to AA may be a fail-safe mechanism that we can access in cases of AA starvation, which could have happened in the past if game or fish were not available for an extended period. There is little question that AA is an EFA for infants and growing children, and for other groups, including diabetics. Many researchers, myself included, think that AA is an EFA for everybody, and that vegan diets threaten the long-term intellectual development of humans.

Arachidonic Acid (AA)

David F. Horrobin, Ph.D., of Scotia Pharmaceuticals in England, gives a saner perspective to the popular notion that arachidonic acid (AA) is a "bad player."

"AA comprises 5 to 15 percent of the fatty acids in cell membranes, and anything present at that level just can't be bad for us!" Dr. Horrobin said. "AA is critical to our health in a number of ways, and thus the body tends to hold on to it. The idea that high intakes of n-3 PUFA will quantitatively 'kick out' AA from cell membranes is incorrect, misleading, and potentially dangerous. AA doesn't leave its position readily, and shouldn't. It takes very large unphysiological intakes of mainly n-3 LC-PUFA to do this. Early studies on cardiovascular disease and supplemental n-3 LC-PUFA (fish oil) were all positive, but some later studies have not been; this may be because these long-term studies did manage to reduce n-6 PUFA too much. Balance between n-3 and n-6 is always the key, and this applies to AA as well."

N-3 PUFA

The n-3 LC-PUFA derivatives of LNA are docosahexaenoic acid (DHA) and eicosapentaenoic acid (EPA). The conversion of LNA to EPA and finally DHA is slow and inefficient in many species, especially humans. The conversion of LNA all the way to DHA may also be a fail-safe mechanism that we can access in cases of DHA or EPA starvation. Perhaps 1 percent of LNA is converted to DHA, unless a person has had a long-term deficiency of n-3 PUFA. When the deficiency is corrected, conversion again slows. Most LNA in the diet is burned for energy. Supplemental LNA in the form of flaxseed or flaxseed oil usually increases plasma EPA two- to fivefold, but does not significantly increase DHA levels. For example, in a 1996 study, 4 weeks of flaxseed oil supplementation increased

LNA in blood plasma cells threefold and EPA by a factor of 2.3, but did not raise DHA levels. Fish oil supplementation for the following 4 weeks dramatically increased both EPA and DHA. In a 1999 study by Neil Mann and others in Melbourne, Australia, lean red meat raised DHA levels in men on mixed diets more than flax oil did in men on vegan diets.

In contrast to LA, LNA is not enriched in organs, and is present in storage fat at only 0.2–0.6 percent. The use of LNA-rich vegetable oils does not appear to produce clinical deficiencies of n-3 PUFA in normal adults. But it is questionable whether LNA-rich vegetable oils alone can correct severe deficiencies or metabolic abnormalities.

LC-PUFA Control the Growth of Intellect

The phrase "fathead" may sound like an insult, but it's quite literally true. Not counting water, which makes up the overwhelming majority of our whole body, the dry weight of our brains is over 60 percent fat. Some of this fat is saturated, and some is polyunsaturated. What's really important is that our central nervous system *does not use* LA and LNA, only their LC-PUFA derivatives.

The LC-PUFA in our brains and spinal cords are made up of about a 1:1 ratio of AA to DHA. This 1:1 ratio in fact, is characteristic of all mammals. In 42 different mammal species studied in depth, the PUFA content of the brains was very similar, with the n-6 to n-3 ratio in the range 1–2:1. The PUFA found in the brains of all the mammals (humans included) were AA, DHA, and small amounts of the intermediate n-6 LC-PUFA metabolite docosatetraenoic acid.

Although the brains of mammals all contain similar ratios of LC-PUFA, human brains are much larger with respect to our body weights. A rhino, for example has a huge brain, but it has an even huger body. The ratio of its brain weight to its body weight is very, very small. For example, a young rhino grows very fast, reaching 1 ton at age 4. A human child weighs about 40 pounds at the same age, but a much higher percentage of that 40 pounds is brain tissue. Our brains also have a more sophisticated and diverse regional organization than do the brains of any other mammals. Adult humans devote about 20 percent of their total energy intake to running the brain, a figure much higher than that for other animals.

Now our ancestors' total percentage of calories from fat is not considered to have exceeded 30–40 percent—but they did not eat fat-free diets either! On the contrary, we are likely to owe our intellect to the fact that we found direct dietary sources of AA and DHA. The lean game meat, fish, and shell-fish we ate were low in overall fat, but rich in AA and DHA in a balanced form. The huge difference between game meat and modern supermarket meat may be a reason why low- to moderate-fat diets rich in *lean* beef or fish *do not* raise choles-terol or increase plaque accumulation in the arteries. In fact, diets with two or more fish meals per week have been shown to significantly reduce the risk for cardiovascular disease.

The huge difference between the intellect of a cow and that of a human is unquestionably due to our adoption of first scavenging and then hunting. Fat from fish and meat was the "brain-specific" nutrient that allowed us to hugely increase the size of our brains without hugely increasing the size of our bodies.

Food Sources of PUFA

The head of the n-6 family is linoleic acid (LA). Significant LA is found in flax, pumpkin, hemp, sun-flower, sesame, grape, and cotton seeds, and in walnuts, corn, peanuts, soybeans, pecans, pistachios, almonds, wheat germ, safflower, and rice bran. The n-6 PUFA derivatives of linoleic acid are gamma-linolenic acid (GLA) and arachidonic acid (AA). Significant GLA is found in evening primrose, borage, and black currant seed oils. AA is widely available in meat, eggs, seafood, and dairy products. AA is sometimes *too* common in Western diets, and it is not supplemented except on rare occasions, such as infant or tube feeding. Growing children, however, should never be denied food sources of AA, because they need it to construct the brain, nervous system, and internal organs.

The head of the n-3 family is alpha-linolenic acid (LNA). LNA is found in significant quantities in flax, mustard, rape (canola), and hemp seeds, and walnuts and soybeans. It is also found at very low levels in green leafy vegetables. Oils containing significant amounts of LNA should be consumed cold-pressed and unrefined. They are not suitable for stove-top cooking or deep frying, only for use as salad oils or in baking. Both high n-3 and, to a lesser extent, n-6, PUFA oils and foods are highly perishable and are quickly destroyed by heat and light. They need to be stored in the dark under refrigeration. Flaxseed oil is the best source of LNA, and is a good source of LA also. Refined, processed canola and soybean oils from the supermarket (or even a health food store!) are *not* good sources of LNA, since LNA may be destroyed during processing.

N-3 LC-PUFA derivatives of LNA are docosahexaenoic acid (DHA) and eicosapentaenoic acid (EPA). These two fatty acids are found in quantity mainly in cold-water fatty marine fish, including salmon, herring, eel, sardines, fresh tuna, mackerel, sturgeon, bluefish, and halibut. Fish such as menhaden and bream from warmer marine waters, and whitefish and trout from fresh water, also contain significant EPA and DHA. In fact, all fish and shellfish contain these LC-PUFA to some degree.

Balanced PUFA Intake Is Critical

Many people supplement or eat PUFA but derive little benefit. Why? They may be consuming poor-quality supplements or highly processed oils. Or their intake of n-6 and n-3 PUFA needs to be balanced. Since n-6 PUFA are far more prevalent in typical foods, many people have adequate or high intakes of n-6, but inadequate n-3 intakes. LA is normally greater than 85 percent of our total dietary PUFA. This high amount of LA is due to the prevalence in our food supply of nuts and agricultural oils such as corn, soybean, peanut, sunflower, safflower, and cottonseed. Our n-3 intake is further reduced by an average intake of over 13 grams per day of *trans*-fats in the North American diet. Remember as well that today's foods are either stripped of PUFA or their balance of fats is wanting.

Dietary PUFA balance is thought to be necessary because n-6 and n-3 fats compete for the same enzymes when our bodies metabolize them. In other words, the enzymes that convert the LA and LNA to their respective derivatives are used for both n-6 and n-3 fats, so that too much of one type of PUFA blocks the absorption or metabolism of the other. However, since we have already found that very little PUFA is actually converted, this can't be the only reason.

More importantly, PUFA balance is required to balance our eicosanoid hormone production, and for insulin to act effectively. High, unbalanced intakes of n-6 PUFA and SFA play a role in the development of diabetes, cancer, chronic inflammatory conditions, and other diseases. Furthermore, humans evolved with relatively low n-6 to n-3 ratios in the diet, and it must be assumed that this balancing effect alone provides benefit. It remains to be proven that unbalanced intakes of any type of fat, and in particular n-6 PUFA, are *not* harmful to humans, not vice versa. We already know, for example, that high unbalanced intakes of SFA and *trans*-fats can significantly increase our risk for diabetes and cardiovascualar disease, and that high unbalanced intakes of LA may increase our risk for cancer.

Our evolutionary diet had a low to moderate amount of fat, and this fat was balanced between natural, unprocessed PUFA, MUFA, and SFA. We evolved eating about a 1:1 ratio of n-6 to n-3. Our current high intake of n-6 polyunsaturated fat, especially in the form of linoleic acid, is unprecedented in human history and prehistory. In most cases, our n-6 to n-3 ratio is on the order of 25–50:1.

In contrast, current dietary guidelines set by U.S., Canadian, and European government health agencies for the *overall ratio* of dietary n-6 to n-3 PUFA range from 4–10:1. Ratios from 4:1 to 1:1 are advocated by many researchers who have examined the fatty acid compositions of the internal organs and brains of man and other higher mammals. Human brain tissue (and that of other mammals) contains an n-6 to n-3 ratio of around 1:1. The ratio in most other cells in the body is 3–5:1. At a minimum, the n-6 to n-3 ratio should be kept in the 5:1 to 1:1 range during the first two years of life, when rapid brain and nervous system development occurs. Human breast milk, an excellent reference standard for our health, normally contains a 4–5:1 ratio.

Please see page 216 for leading PUFA and flaxseed researcher Dr. Stephen C. Cunnane's view on flaxseed and n-3 PUFA in the diet.

PUFA and Diabetes

Cell membranes that are flexible have more and better insulin receptors, and allow for better glucose metabolism. PUFA help make cell membranes flexible, whereas SFA make them stiffer. This means that a diet high in saturated fats or hydrogenated fats can cause or contribute to diabetes. Conversely, a diet low in overall fat but with a relatively high ratio of PUFA to SFA helps prevent diabetes. Most important are n-3 PUFA. Many studies have shown that the cell membranes of diabetics have an abnormal fat composition. The membranes are too stiff, and the levels of LC-PUFA are too low. This does not mean that diabetes can't develop if membrane flexibility is normal, but rather that PUFA metabolism plays a greater or lesser role in diabetes depending on an individual's diet and genetics.

The hormone insulin *stimulates,* and the hormone glucagon *inhibits,* the enzyme system that converts PUFA to LC-

PUFA. The balance of these hormones thus dramatically influences which PUFA are available for incorporation into cell membranes. As was the case with obesity, the situation is a feedback loop, because the fatty acid composition of membrane lipids also influences the action of insulin. Experiments have shown that increasing membrane flexibility by feeding higher dietary levels of PUFA increases the number of insulin receptors and insulin action.

The Type II diabetes condition may be the *result* of accumulating membrane abnormalities. And we must look to recent changes in our diet to see if perhaps we've been eating foods that could adversely affect the flexibility of our cell membranes.

Insulin Resistance and Skeletal Muscles

Diets too high in SFA, *trans*-fats, and n-6 PUFA adversely affect insulin efficiency and glucose response. Skeletal muscles, the major users of glucose in the body, are constantly stimulated by insulin. Numerous experiments have determined that high-fat diets increase the accumulation of storage fat in skeletal muscles. In a steak or slice of prime rib, this storage fat within the muscle is known as marbling, but such fat is a common feature in human muscles also. This marbled fat leads directly to insulin resistance in the individual muscles. Not surprisingly, most of this fat is SFA. Losing some of this fat improves or helps prevent diabetes. In addition, if a significant percentage of n-3 PUFA is substituted for other fat in the diet, insulin resistance can be improved or prevented.

Is Fish Oil Safe for People with Diabetes?

Concerns that fish oil or other n-3 LC-PUFA supplementation might cause elevated glucose levels in diabetics, by reducing insulin secretion, have not been confirmed by recent research. A 1997 multicenter double-blind study on

935 subjects found that plasma triglycerides (triacylglyc-erols) decreased up to 21.5 percent with modest supple-mentation of n-3 LC-PUFA. In addition to high blood triglycerides, 55 percent of the subjects had diabetes or impaired glucose tolerance, and 68 percent had high blood pressure.

Subjects were given 1,530 mg of EPA and 1,050 mg of DHA daily for 2 months, which was then decreased to 1,020 mg of EPA and 700 mg of DHA daily for the fol-lowing 4 months. Placebo subjects received olive oil. No adverse effects on blood sugar control or blood pressure were recorded, and those with diabetes had proportion-ally greater decreases in triglycerides and increases in HDL cholesterol than those without diabetes.

Holistic Treatment Supplements

Mark Swanson, N.D., of the Naturopathic Wellness & Diagnosis Center in Sequim, Washington, uses supple-ments in his natural holistic treatment program for dia-betes.

Dr. Swanson said, "Though supplement needs are indi-vidualized to each patient, the following are among my most prescribed for diabetes prevention and treatment."

High-potency multivitamin/mineral, with at least the following per day in divided doses: vitamin C, 1000 mg; vitamin E, 200 IU; 25 mg each vitamin B_1, B_3, B_6; 200 mcg B_{12}; 400 mcg folic acid; 150 mcg chromium; 150 mcg selenium; 200 mg calcium; 200 mg magnesium; zinc, 30 mg; natural beta-carotene, 10,000 iu; vitamin D, 200 IU.

Additional Supplementation

Magnesium glycinate or citrate, 600 mg per day
Vitamin C (mixed ascorbates), 2–4 grams per day
Vitamin E (natural source tocopherol), 400 IU per day
Vitamin E (natural source succinate), 400 IU per day

Chromium (picolinate or polynicotinate), up to 1,000 mcg daily

Mixed natural carotenoids, 25,000–50,000 IU per day

Lycopene, 10 mg per day

Alpha lipoic acid, 300–600 mg per day

Tocotrienols, 25–200 mg per day

Folic acid, 400 mcg day

Garlic (deodorized), one tablet per meal

Conjugated linoleic acid (Tonalin brand), 1,000 mg three times daily with meals

- Vanadyl sulfate can also significantly improve glucose tolerance, but should be taken only under physician supervision.
- *Gymnema sylvestre*: Though this herb is reported to improve glucose control, Dr. Swanson has not found it of much help in his patients.
- Prickly pear cactus (nopal) can also lower fasting blood sugar. It's best to eat the whole cooked vegetable rather than take supplements.

Diabetes and High-MUFA (Olive Oil) Diets

High-MUFA diets, such as the olive oil–based Mediterranean diet, are potentially beneficial for people with diabetes. Here, calories from MUFA are substituted for some of the calories in the diet provided previously by carbohydrates and sometimes SFA. This only works, however, if the MUFA is substituted isocalorically for the carbohydrates or SFA. *Isocalorically* means that the calorie switch is equal, and since MUFA have 9 calories per gram, but carbohydrates have 4 calories per gram, less volume of food is consumed. If the diet has fat of any type simply added to it, there is no benefit, and there might even be the detrimental effect of weight gain.

In these approaches, MUFA is burned off for energy. It is not provided to be stored or to improve the flexibility of cell membranes, such as with LC-PUFA. The underlying assumption in high-MUFA diets is that structural PUFA are not deficient.

It's important to make the distinction between fat that is either stored or burned for energy and structural fat. In the sections above, we have discussed structural fat as contained in the cell membranes of insulin-sensitive tissues. This is an entirely different issue from what food is being burned for energy. The Modern Evolutionary Diet, my best choice for diabetes, even meshes closely with many aspects of the Mediterranean diet, since both emphasize lots of fruits, vegetables, and nuts, less refined carbohydrate, and more whole foods. However, I put more emphasis on lean protein and do not recommend basing diets on pasta, grains, and beans.

Many people with diabetes may be better off eating MUFA in exchange for carbohydrate, but this alone will not prevent or reverse diabetes. The question relating to the fat content of hunter-gatherer diets and the origin of diabetes is not simply: "Which dietary fats can best ameliorate existing diabetes?" More importantly, the question is: "Is the profound loss of n-3 LC-PUFA or imbalance in triglyceride types in the current Western diet a potentially preventable *cause* of diabetes?"

To answer this question, we must consider the potential effects on structural fat of a lifetime of consuming dietary fats composed mainly of SFA, LA, and *trans*-fats. A 1997 study found that *trans*-MUFA were not beneficial for diabetics. Sixteen obese diabetes patients were fed 20 percent of calories from either *trans*-MUFA, *cis*-MUFA (oleic acid, such as from olive oil), or SFA in a diet with 30 percent of calories from fat overall. Each diet was eaten for 6 weeks. Both SFA and *trans*-MUFA increased the insulin levels after meals, but *cis*-MUFA had no effect. Blood glucose and triglycerides were not significantly different in any of the groups, which may indicate reduced insulin sensitivity in the SFA and *trans*-MUFA groups.

Both the quantity and type of fat ingested influence insulin sensitivity. Since skeletal muscle is the largest user of glucose in the body, maintaining a high lean-fat tissue ratio is an overall recommendation for diabetes prevention and reversal. In addition, reducing SFA and n-6 PUFA, while increasing n-3 PUFA, is recommended. Some percentage of n-3 PUFA should be from n-3 LC-PUFA, since there is variation in PUFA intake and metabolism among populations.

PUFA Supplementation Guidelines for Diabetes

In the basic supplement plan of my diet, I recommend supplementing PUFA precursors and LC-PUFA derivatives simultaneously. This approach maximizes potential benefits, while minimizing potential risks. I also recommend this approach for treating both Types I and II diabetes.

Since our diets often are already overly rich in n-6 PUFA, mostly in the form of LA, oils used for effective nutritional supplementation must be very rich in n-3. Otherwise, we will simply be providing even more LA to our bodies—bodies already overloaded with LA, and with a likely result of more weight gain! A good rule of thumb for everyone here is to supplement PUFA in a 1:1 n-6 to n-3 ratio.

Supplementation per Day for Both Types I and II Diabetes

3,000 mg evening primrose oil (1,300 mg 3 times per day is fine also; some manufacturers use this size).

3,000 mg fish or marine algae oil.

Do not totally avoid AA in the form of animal fat.

2–4 teaspoons cold-pressed unrefined flaxseed oil or Essential Balance oil.

Notes

1. Children 4–12 use one-half the adult dose; under 4 use one-third the adult dose. There is no harm with extra! Children with allergies, eczema, psoriasis, chronic dermatitis, asthma, learning disabilities, autism, candida infections, or other conditions that warrant PUFA supplementation should up their dosage one age group.

2. For adults with chronic skin conditions, allergies, arthritis, PMS, or other conditions that warrant GLA supplementation, there is no harm in doubling the dose of evening primrose or borage oils.
3. Evening primrose oil can help halt the progression of diabetic nerve disease (diabetic neuropathy). Increase evening primrose or borage oil intake to 4–6 grams per day to help prevent neuropathy.
4. You may increase the dose of the fish oil if your diet has been deficient in n-3 PUFA for some time, unless you are on blood-thinning medications or equivalent natural products. If this is the case, check with your doctor before exceeding 2,000 mg.

PART
TWO

The Modern Evolutionary Diet Plan

6

The Modern Evolutionary Diet Plan Guidelines

The Modern Evolutionary Diet is designed to help you lose fat, prevent chronic disease, improve energy levels, and develop healthy eating habits that you can use your whole life. It is also *specifically* a diet for prevention and management of diabetes. The diet is primarily focused on permanent body fat loss, but it can also be used by those who wish to maintain their present weight, or even gain weight. Recommendations for maintaining and gaining weight are given in Chapter 8, but I recommend that you don't skip ahead, because the groundwork for understanding those recommendations starts right here.

Even if you have been eating a junk food diet and are loath to give it up, you can start to improve your diet and health by easing into the Modern Evolutionary Diet. Try it some days of the week, and do whatever you usually do on the other days. In doing so, you may discover some new things about how your body reacts to different foods and eating habits. Know also that a properly nourished and exercised body usually responds to a medication, be it herbal or pharmaceutical, more quickly and with a better chance of the desired result. This can result in your using only the minimum dosage of a drug, which is safer and reduces potential side effects. If the medication you are taking is for controlling diabetes, you can look to a brighter future. The Modern Evolutionary Diet with exercise and natural supplements will nearly or completely eliminate your need for the drug.

Remember, too, the Modern Evolutionary Diet is not difficult, expensive, or troublesome to follow, and does not require special foods or preparation techniques. If you are willing, and really want to prevent or reverse diabetes, all you need to do is open your mind and work a little.

Food Allergies

If, in addition to chronic weight problems, you have migraines, other severe headaches, fluid retention, asthma, eczema, psoriasis, gastrointestinal problems, chronic hives, adult acne or rashes, chronic nasal and sinus congestion or infections, abnormally bad PMS, chronic fatigue, rheumatoid arthritis, fibromyalgia, irritability, or any other chronic condition that has not been resolved despite numerous attempts, you may have undiagnosed food allergies.

If you have food allergies, no diet will ever succeed until you identify the offending foods and remove them from your meals. (After you are well, in most cases you can rotate such foods on a limited basis.) Nobody can really help you if you don't take care of this issue. In your case, comprehensive food allergy testing is as vital as an X-ray is to diagnose a broken bone. If this sounds like you, part of your initial effort with the Modern Evolutionary Diet should include your reading of Chapter 11. It would be unfortunate if you set yourself up for failure by designing your version of the diet plan based strongly on foods that you are allergic to. If you do have delayed-onset food allergies, the chances that you will indeed set your diet up that way are very good.

Fats

To ensure success with the diet, we also need to reemphasize the crucial distinction between structural fat and storage fat. Fat nutrition is complex, and is often poorly or incorrectly explained in too many nutrition and diet books. Fat nutrition is also critically important to the health of people with diabetes. Structural fat—containing polyunsaturated fat (PUFA), also known as the essential fatty acids—is critical to our health, because it is a major component of all cell membranes, internal organs, and brain and nervous tissue. Losing body fat *does not* mean losing or degrading our structural fat. Storage fat is largely saturated fat. Our ancestors needed to carry around excess food for emergencies. We have kitchens and supermarkets to store food now, so we don't need much storage fat—but we continue to accumulate it! Losing body fat *does* mean losing storage fat.

While cutting the percentage of calories from fat in your diet can really help you lose fat and decrease your risk for chronic disease, there is a point of diminishing returns. Remember that there are two families of PUFA, n-6 and n-3. Each of these are essential, and they are not interchangeable. We operate best when the ratio of n-6 to n-3 PUFA is in the range 9:1 to 1:1. We operate poorly or not at all when PUFA are deficient or greatly imbalanced, regardless of the other fats that might be included in the diet.

Unlike carbohydrate, fat is an essential nutrient. You can set yourself up for failure in your version of the diet plan if you try to cut the percentage of calories from fat down to 5–15 percent, as many popular diets recommend. If you starve yourself of PUFA, either by eating too little fat or the wrong kind of fat, you will never be able to stick to a fat loss diet. Fatty foods will call to you day and night, until you break down and overeat them. If these foods are typical diet busters like potato chips and pepperoni pizza, they won't provide you with much of the balanced PUFA that your body needs, so that you'll repeat the cycle day after day. You can't fool your ancient body—it's looking for specific nutrients and will signal "keep eating" as long as they're lacking.

Eating adequate, balanced, unrefined PUFA is *the only way* to permanently cure a persistent craving for fatty foods!

Guideline 1

The percentages of calories in the Modern Evolutionary Diet are 20 percent from fat, 30–35 percent from protein, and 45–50 percent from carbohydrate. Fat has more than twice as many calories per unit weight as protein and carbohydrate, and so is a more concentrated source of energy. Read the labels on foods to see what the fat, protein, and carbohydrate breakdown is.

1 gram protein = 4 calories
1 gram carbohydrate = 4 calories
1 gram fat = 9 calories
1 gram alcohol = 7 calories (approximately 2 ml of 100 proof)

Guideline 2

Limit carbohydrate consumption to fruits and starchy vegetables such as peas, corn, lima beans, winter squash, potatoes, and beets. Eat no pasta, bread, noodles, macaroni, rice, cereal, or crackers. Eat absolutely no sugar or sugary foods, keeping in mind that the worst food ever invented is the doughnut. Don't drink fruit juices, except a little in blender drinks—eat only the whole fruit. Eat one serving of bread or cereal for an occasional treat, but the less the better. Unlike many diets, we don't bother counting the carbohydrates of any nonstarchy vegetables. The small amount of carbohydrate in an onion, for example, does not count toward your daily percentage of calories from carbohydrate.

The simplest carbohydrate rule for the fastest weight loss: "If it's sugar-sweet or made of wheat, don't eat!"

Guideline 3

Don't eat meals or snacks composed mainly or wholly of carbohydrate foods, especially at breakfast and late at night. Meals and snacks need to be a balance of protein, carbohydrate, and fat. Don't be fooled by fat-free cookies, rice cakes, and other such snack foods. Can you really eat only two rice cakes and feel satisfied? Eating protein, fat, and a little carbohydrate at each meal or large snack is a good policy for controlling hunger, as well as blood sugar, if you are diabetic. Pure carbohydrate snacks and meals leave us begging for more, or hungry in a few hours, and are never recommended for diabetics.

Guideline 4

Never reach for starch or sugar when you are hungry. When you are really hungry, eat plain low-fat protein and water first, or a food such as yogurt, cottage cheese, or a high-protein sports nutrition bar. Eat only when you are truly hungry — don't make a habit of eating "preemptively" to prevent yourself from being hungry. The first week is always the hardest—it gets much easier after that.

Guideline 5

Eat copious quantities of fresh, preferably raw, nonstarchy vegetables (first choice) and fruits (second choice). Don't count vegetable calories or carbohydrates, except for avocados, potatoes, sweet potatoes, corn, and other such starchy vegetables. Count calories and carbohydrates in all fruits. Don't be obsessive about counting calories in fruits and vegetables, though. If you stop eating sugar, grains, and most fat, you hardly need to count calories at all!

Guideline 6

Do not drink alcohol. Fats have 9 calories per gram and alcohol has 7. Weight loss is next to impossible with any drinking, unless you are a serious alcoholic, in which case you live mostly on whatever alcoholic drink you consume. Alcohol, like refined sugars and starches, forces you to cannibalize your body's nutrient stores just to metabolize it.

Guideline 7

Always consume your daily protein requirement. Your daily protein requirement is the anchor of the diet. *You cannot thrive without meeting this requirement, only just survive.* When I do a personal consultation, I calculate protein requirements for the client. In this text, we'll have to work together to make an estimate. If you know your lean body mass, that is best. It can be measured at health clubs and by some sports oriented physicians or nutritionists. Many fitness books also give tables for calculating lean body mass and protein requirements. However, by consulting the box titled "Estimating Your Daily Protein Requirement," you can make an estimate that is quite accurate enough for the purpose of this diet.

To determine the protein content of packaged foods, read the Nutrition Facts table on the label. A good guide is that one 6-ounce can of tuna packed in water has around 30 grams of protein; one heaping scoop of protein powder (28 grams or 1 ounce) usually has about 20 grams. Protein foods such as fat-free or low-fat hot dogs and deli meats are a good way to start, if you have difficulty estimating the protein content of foods, because they come in standardized servings. Keep in mind that these products are precooked, and so have much less water than raw meats. The protein and calorie content per unit weight of deli-sliced turkey is similar to that of cooked sliced skinless turkey breast, not raw turkey.

Guideline 8

Omit or strongly limit fresh cuts of beef, pork, and lamb until you have lost one-third to one-half the weight you wish

Aubrey Hampton's Story

A committed vegan for many years, eating mainly carbohydrate foods, Aubrey Hampton, of Aubrey Organics Inc., the manufacturer of the only 100 percent natural organic line of hair, skin, and cosmetic products, found that he had to change his diet to control his diabetes.

"As a Type II diabetic, I'm a bit unusual—I'm not over-weight," Hampton said. "But diet has been the key to reducing my medication and keeping my blood sugar stabilized. I find that a high-protein diet and food sup-plements have been very helpful. Often I'll have bacon and eggs for breakfast (organic, of course), with half a grapefruit. Lunch is a salad or perhaps some leftovers from last night's dinner. Frequently I'll have a glass of champagne or red wine with dinner, which is often chicken or beef with fresh vegetables. I love pasta, but I find I do better if I only eat it once a week or so, since it tends to raise my blood sugar the next morning. As for nutritional supplements, I'm prone to bad colds, so vita-min C supplementation is essential to me. I take at least three grams of buffered C per day. I also take 1,000 IU mixed tocopherols of vitamin E, grapeseed extract (phy-tosomes), milk thistle (to counteract that wine!), alpha lipoic acid, quercetin, and bilberry.

"I've recently started taking a product from Enzymatic Therapy called Doctor's Choice for Diabetics, which con-tains vitamins, minerals, and herbs especially beneficial for diabetics. [The ingredients include chromium picoli-nate, vitamin E, B_{12}, B_6, folic acid, magnesium, seleni-um, vanadyl sulfate, fenugreek, bilberry, bitter melon, and *Gymnema sylvestre*—all of which are mentioned in this book.] My blood sugar has been lower since I started to take it; I don't know for sure that this is due to the supplements, but they certainly seem to have helped. I also take a tablespoon of organic flaxseed oil every day without fail. It keeps my hands soft. Since starting this regimen, my cholesterol has dropped 20 points and I've lost 5 pounds. My doctor just shakes her head and wants to know what I'm doing. I know I should exercise more, but as head of Aubrey Organics, I get a workout keeping track of my products and the stores that sell them."

Estimating Your Daily Protein Requirement

If you have been lean or at normal weight for most of your life and are just trying to get rid of excess pounds that have crept on over time through aging, pregnancy, or inactivity, do the following: Choose your ideal weight in pounds, that is, the weight that you would like to arrive at. Don't lie to yourself—pick the weight you used to be when you were a young adult, or perhaps 10–20 pounds less. Then subtract 10 percent for men and 20 percent for women. This weight is a good estimate of your lean body mass.

However, if you are very heavy or obese and have been heavy or struggling with your weight most of your life, choose the ideal weight in pounds that you think you can reach to be considerably lighter and healthier. Subtract 15 percent for men and 25 percent for women. This is a good estimate of your lean body mass.

Next, multiply your lean body mass by one of the activity factors below. If you think you are between categories, you can use 0.65, for example, instead of 0.6 or 0.7. Slight overestimation is better than underestimation. The number you get is the grams of protein you need to consume every day. To lose fat, try to eat just the protein you need every day, not more and not less. Protein is not stored up one day and consumed the next. If you do not eat adequate daily protein, your body will cannibalize its own muscle structure. If you eat far more protein than you need, it is just excess calories. However, excess protein calories are less likely to be stored as fat than excess carbohydrate calories and especially excess fat calories. If you are diabetic, you can replace carbohydrate calories with protein calories above your requirement and achieve very good success in controlling blood sugar.

Activity Factors

0.5 Sedentary, no formal sports training or regular activity.

0.6 Light fitness training such as walking or a job that requires work on your feet.

0.7 Moderate exercise or team sports participation, 3–4 days per week.

0.8 Daily aerobic or moderate weight training. Also physical jobs such as construction, landscaping, demolition, shipping and delivery.

0.9 Heavy weight training or extremely physical jobs such as ski instructor, lumberjack, refuse pickup.

1.0 Heavy weight training along with intense aerobic workout. Semipro or pro-athletic team training or other elite competitive training. Use 1.0 if you want to gain a lot of muscle also.

Note: Pregnant or nursing women, add 0.2 to your factor.

Note: Diabetics with confirmed or suspected renal complications (kidney disease or dysfunction) or Type I diabetics on protein-restricted diets may not be able to scale up protein intake with activity factors. If this is your situation, use your doctor's dietary recommendations, and at a maximum, stick to the activity factor for sedentary individuals. If you do need to restrict protein, it is in your best interest to have your lean body mass measured accurately by a professional, and to eat proteins of high quality or biological values, so that you can be very precise in your protein intake.

Protein Choices

Here are my suggestions for lean protein choices. They are listed in order of highest quality to lowest quality, but this is not exact. All choices are reasonably good, and you can mix them up in any variety that suits you.

1. Cold-processed whey peptide protein powder
2. Egg white, egg white protein powder, or liquid protein
3. Fish
4. Shellfish
5. Skinless poultry
6. Game meats such as venison or buffalo
7. Very lean red meat
8. Whole eggs
9. Low-fat luncheon meats, hot dogs, etc.
10. Fat-free or low-fat cottage cheese
11. Other dairy products
12. Tofu and other soy protein products

to lose, and then eat these at a maximum of two or three times per week. Some exceptions might be made for extra lean beef jerky and low-fat sausages, for example. However, be flexible if there is no alternative while you are traveling, doing business, or dining out. A pork tenderloin or lean steak and a big salad are much better than pasta. There's no problem with animal protein *per se,* as long as it is consumed in moderation and is free of excess fat.

Guideline 9

Limit or omit soups (especially canned), stews, preprepared one-dish meals, and most casseroles and long-cooked foods. *The more plain, raw food, the better.* Separating the parts of a meal into a meat or fish serving, salad or green vegetable serving, starch serving, and dessert serving is the best way to plan family meals. This helps you pick out what is protein, fat, and carbohydrate, and makes sure that you don't eat something like a huge serving of noodles with a few pieces of chicken and carrots decorating them, as is the case in most canned chicken noodle soups. If you like to cook, you can easily make stews and soups in the Modern Evolutionary Diet way with the recipe suggestions in Chapter 10.

Guideline 10

Sip plain water all day. You should have to urinate every two hours while you are awake. The time spent in the bathroom will pay you back more than double by increased alertness. Many of us are walking around constantly in a state of mild dehydration, and concentration on a task is the first thing to go. This is especially important if you have asthma, allergies, constipation, or chronic indigestion.

Guideline 11

Eat cooked dried beans for a treat only if you like them. *Beans count as a carbohydrate food, not a protein food.* Use them as a side dish or condiment, not as a protein source. There's no need to make a special effort to eat beans when egg whites, tuna fish, and protein powder are cheap and readily available. Beans are poor-quality protein and extremely high in carbohydrates.

You never combine beans and grains for (supposedly) balanced protein in the Modern Evolutionary Diet. Humans evolved completely in the absence of these foods. Eating these foods is a semistarvation subsistence agriculture eating strategy, not a strategy for losing fat, gaining muscle, or preventing or reversing diabetes.

Guideline 12

What I said about beans applies to soybeans as well. While some foods fortified with soy protein isolate can have value, soy protein is of poorer quality than animal protein and highly overpromoted. Like beans, tofu, soy milks and cheeses, and other bean curd products contain quite a bit of carbohydrate and sometimes fat, along with the protein. In the United

States and Canada, ounce for ounce, canned tuna and cottage cheese are much cheaper sources of protein than tofu, and taste a lot better, too! Soy protein may be needed in the diet in case of food allergies, but is usually not eaten for this reason. It takes 5,000 calories of rice or 1833 calories of beans to get 100 grams of protein. Pure protein has only 400 calories in 100 grams. So you be the judge of which choice will help you lose fat.

Guideline 13

Avoid refined and processed carbohydrates and fats as much as possible. This includes mainly pastries, cookies, cakes, candies, junk foods, and fried foods. If you see partially hydrogenated or hydrogenated oil on the label, don't buy it! If the food comes in a box or crimped shelf wrapper, think it over carefully and read the Nutrition Facts! Virtually everything you eat should be perishable. If you are dying for a high-fat food, choose nuts, cheese, steak, whole eggs, or pork chops. Do not reach for snack chips, fries, candy, doughnuts, or pastries.

Guideline 14

Keep fiber intake high, especially soluble fiber. Eating plenty of fruits and vegetables will do this easily, and special fiber supplements such as flaxseed meal and citrus pectin can really help. Nobody needs to eat bran cereal or oat bran bread to get enough fiber. Since we evolved completely in the absence of agriculture, we did not have these foods in our diet until very recently. To get fiber, our ancestors ate lots of fibrous green plant foods and some nuts and wild seeds.

Guideline 15

Dieting is doomed to fail if you don't get enough of the nutrients you need. I don't recommend any weight loss diet unless it includes an intelligent and balanced basic supplement plan as well. Supplements are not a substitute for a diet of healthful foods—they are simply one part of it! Supple-ments can help you avoid some of the initial fatigue that may be associated with reducing your food intake, and are particularly important if your health is already compromised by diabetes.

Guideline 16

For dieting, it is better to pick one day a week to overeat or drink alcohol significantly than to eat or drink a little too much every day. Prior to agriculture and food storage, humans commonly lived in a feast or famine mode, periodically stuffing themselves when food was plentiful. We seem to do fine and not gain weight eating an occasional Thanksgiving dinner, but 200–500 extra calories each day slowly but surely put on the pounds. In addition, with 7 calories per gram, even moderate daily alcohol consumption is enough to prevent the body from losing fat and to deplete the body of vitamins and minerals.

Taking a day or two off the Modern Evolutionary Diet per week is an excellent strategy for easing into the diet, and for sticking to it for the long haul. You can, for example, take yourself or your family out to an all-you-can-eat spaghetti night at your local Italian restaurant and eat all you want. Or perhaps Sunday is your day to watch football, drink beer, and eat chips and burgers. Do what you want on Sunday, just pull in the reins on Monday.

Guideline 17

If you always cheat on something, simply do not purchase it. You are in control at the store. Reserve it for your day off or other special occasions and go out for it. Alternatively, tell yourself that you can indeed have it anytime you want, but you must go out to pick it up. Resist the temptation to buy Oreos, Girl Scout cookies, snack chips, and so on for visiting kids or friends. They are horrid nutritionally, so you're not doing them any favors if you serve them. These products are loaded with *trans*-fats, preservatives, and refined carbohydrates. Home-made cookies are much better, if you must have cookies!

Guideline 18

Body fat loss is best accomplished with a combination of diet and exercise. The benefits of diet and exercise are synergistic, both physically and mentally, and nothing succeeds like success. So, get meaningful exercise as often as possible, and do your exercise for an hour or more if you can. You can exercise a little throughout your day by upping your overall pace. If all you can do is walk, then walk. But move on to alternating days walking with days of more strenuous activity. Do all your house and yard work or shopping at breakneck speed, so that you can have more time for your meaningful exercise and get more exercise while you work! Vacuuming or mowing fast, for example, can be real work. The more you get into the diet, the more energy you will have.

Natural Estrogen from Plants

James Duke, Ph.D., author of *The Green Pharmacy*, was promoting the benefits of phytochemicals, herbal alternatives, and functional foods long before most of the rest of us had even heard these phrases, let alone put them into practice! Dr. Duke spends considerable time and effort reminding us that, in our daily meals, we're just scratching the surface of sampling the thousands of edible plants in the world. He also comments that the legume family is very large and that soybeans, while having their good points, are nothing more than average legumes. There is much interest in the phytoestrogenic isoflavone (mainly genistein and diadzein) content of soybeans, and some misguided promoters have stated that soybeans are unique sources of these compounds. Nothing could be farther from the truth.

"Scurfy pea (*Psoralea corylifolia*) proved more than sixty times richer than soy in genistein," Dr. Duke said. "Soybean was by no means highest, as soy scientists had claimed. The data presented below are in descending order of genistein content."

Seed Sample	Genistein (ppm)	Diadzein (ppm)
Psoralea corylifolia	1528.0	539.7
Kudzu root	316.9	949.8
Yellow split pea	45.8	0.4
Black turtle beans	45.1	0.4
Baby lima beans	40.1	0.4
Large lima beans	34.4	0.3
Anasazi beans	29.8	6.5
Red kidney beans	29.3	2.7
Red lentils	25.0	5.2
SOYBEANS	24.1	37.6
Black-eyed peas	23.3	0.3
Pinto beans	22.3	23.2
Mung beans	21.8	0.3
Azuki beans	21.2	4.6
Fava beans	19.9	5.0
Great northern beans	17.7	7.2
Anthyllis vulneraria	3.7	1.8

7

Designing Meals

Refined and processed foods are to be avoided as much as possible. Of the four kinds to be avoided, the first and largest offender is refined grains, followed by refined sugars and corn syrup, hydrogenated fats, and refined and processed proteins.

Refined Grains

If you base your diet on refined grains, you are forcing your body to overeat calories. Obvious refined grains include white flour and white bread. However, most people don't realize that pasta, macaroni, noodles, cream of wheat, pearled barley, many cereals, rice cakes, degerminated corn meal, and white rice are just the same—refined starches. When starting the diet, avoid cereal grains altogether. Later, after some success, choose whole grain versions whenever possible, and eat mostly oatmeal and other porridge grains. Supermarket "whole wheat" sandwich breads, muffins, and bagels have only small amounts of whole wheat flour. Those from specialty bakeries or health food stores may be better, but read the labels! "Wheat flour" on the labels means white flour, not whole wheat. Whole wheat flour must be listed on the labels as "whole wheat flour."

We need to learn to read the Nutrition Facts on labels scrupulously. Many commercial muffins, for example, are over 400 calories each and loaded with fat and sugar, even if they are bran or carrot and marketed as "healthy." A typical, individually wrapped blueberry muffin in my local 7-Eleven store has 420 calories and 20 grams of fat. A 4-ounce square (about four bites) of the carrot bread in the same store has the same calorie content and a whopping 23 grams of fat! Much of this fat is *trans*-fatty acids and saturated fat, and all the sugar is refined.

Refined Sugars and Corn Syrup

The second worst offenders, refined sugars and corn syrup, are included in almost all desserts and sweet foods, commercial baked goods and cereals, and many sauces, dips, fruit juices, and processed meat items. *A high-sugar diet defeats all attempts at fat loss.* Foods such as candy, doughnuts, danishes, and store-bought cookies and cakes are to be avoided in any weight loss diet—even the new fat-free and low-fat versions. They are still junk, and are specially designed by the manufacturers to make you eat without feeling full. If you must have a sweet, rich snack, choose nuts, hot cocoa, cafe latte, pudding, sweetened yogurt, chocolate milk, or a sports nutrition snack bar, instead of cookies, candy, or pastries. Try to get at least some protein in with your sugar!

Sugar consumption must be minimized or reduced in the Modern Evolutionary Diet. On labels this means sugar, sucrose, glucose, corn syrup, corn sweetener, dextrose, fructose, lactose, levulose, maltodextrin, invert sugar, concentrated fruit juice, invertase, sorbitol, xylitol, mannitol, barley malt, malt extract and various syrups and honey. Read labels as much as possible. Seemingly innocuous products such as steak sauce, catsup, pickles, salad dressing, tartar sauce, mustard, salsa, pasta sauce, fruit yogurt, lunch meats, BBQ sauce, crackers, and salty snack foods can have a huge percentage of their calories from sugar! Almost all commercial baked goods and cereals are loaded with sugar. Manufacturers use the cleverest ways they can to disguise the sugar they use. If you learn to read food labels thoroughly, though, you won't be fooled.

Refined sugar has no nutrition. In fact, sugar and alcohol are the best examples of foods for which the body must cannibalize its own stores of vitamins and minerals just to digest. For the rest of your life, after you have lost the weight you want to, try to eat sugar only when it is a small, combined component of foods (for example, muffins, cereals, sports nutrition bars, sweetened yogurts, and fruit salads), and not as candy, cookies, cakes, desserts, frostings, sweet drinks, ice cream, sherbet, or jellies. This advice is part of every dietary recommendation for diabetics.

Sugar makes the blood acidic, and lymphocytes (our white blood cells that attack and kill viruses, bacteria, and other foreign proteins) don't work nearly as effectively when the blood is acidic. Overconsumption of refined sugar is involved in chronic allergies, colds, and ear infections. It is also implicated in high cholesterol levels and heart disease. High intakes of sugar are linked to high cholesterol levels, because they deplete the body's chromium reserves and impair enzyme function, and the sugar metabolites provide the precursor molecules for cholesterol synthesis in the liver. Loading the bloodstream with sugar is also a risk factor for cancer. Cancer cells don't metabolize glucose in the way that normal cells do and tend to consume more glucose than normal cells do. I could add 25 more reasons here, or you can find entire books on this subject in your local health food store or bookstore.

In addition to its immunosuppressive effects, when refined sugar acidifies the blood, other problems occur. Acidic conditions grossly impair muscle and enzyme function, and cause wide fluctuations of blood sugar, so that too much sugar is always directly detrimental to athletic performance. However, high-quality energy replacement drinks used directly after strenuous (and I mean strenuous!) exercise are beneficial. Fructose, for example, is used quickly to replenish glycogen stores in the liver.

Hydrogenated Fats

The third worst offenders are the hydrogenated fats found in nearly all commercial baked goods, shortening, margarine, snack chips and other deep fried foods, and supermarket vegetable oils. Hydrogenated fats are also known as *trans*-fats. Be especially cautious about cookies, crackers, granola bars, and microwave popcorn. Even the reduced-fat versions are filled with hydrogenated fats. Do your own corn popping if you must, and try using butterscotch-flavored Essential Balance Jr. or unrefined flaxseed oil instead of, or mixed with, real butter. Shopping for packaged items and baked goods for your whole family in a health food store or natural foods supermarket is a good idea; however, homemade is an even better idea. Choose naturally low-fat products and prudently add your own healthful fats and spreads, if you like.

Refined and Processed Proteins

Refined and processed proteins are not much of an offender. Certainly, deli slices of precooked maple-glazed turkey are not as healthful as home-cooked sliced turkey breast, but processed proteins in general have more benefits than drawbacks. The benefits of lunch and deli meats, hot dogs, canned tuna, and sausage are that they are convenient, safe, portable, and fast ways to get measured amounts of very low-fat protein. The drawbacks include excess salt, high temperature processing, preservatives, fillers, sugars, and extra water. The fillers, sugars, and extra water can make the protein content per serving of processed meats and seafoods lower than their fresh-cooked equivalents. The best choice is to use these products when necessary, but not exclusively. They can help you learn how much protein a certain amount of food has, and as we shall see, they may also be critical in teaching your children to eat the Modern Evolutionary Diet way.

Certain types of proteins have been super-processed, not to make them super-tasty and bland like white sugar and flour, but rather to make them super-digestible. This includes the whole family of protein powders and weight gainer products that have been traditionally marketed to bodybuilders. Serious bodybuilders and professional athletes have known for years that they need to have protein sources that are (1) very easily digested and assimilated, (2) of highest quality or biological value, (3) highly concentrated and pure, (4) hypoallergenic, (5) very low fat, and (6) available to eat more or less instantly. My first choice is cold-processed ion-exchanged whey peptide protein powder, but egg white protein and whey/egg blends are great also. Tasty liquid proteins in flavors like vanilla and peanut butter are also back on the market now. These products are a cornerstone of the Modern Evolutionary Diet, and the best example of how we use technology to update how our ancestors ate, but not change the basic principles of their diet.

To learn how to use protein powder beyond mixing it in milk, fruit juice, or yogurt, investigate the blender drink recipes in Chapter 10. With my busy schedule, I sometimes live on these, because I will not compromise my nutrition (nor that of my family), no matter how hectic life is. Nothing else is so important; and one of my secrets for being productive while juggling a busy schedule is the Modern Evolutionary Diet.

Fresh Produce

A lack of fresh produce in any diet puts you at a health disadvantage. The diet supplement plan of Chapter 8 gives you the basic vitamins and minerals that are in fruits and vegetables, but there is no substitute for the many complex compounds and fiber found in produce that protect us from a variety of diseases, aid our digestion, and give us energy. *In every single applicable study of chronic disease, the higher the fruit and vegetable consumption, the lower the disease risk.* We are genetically programmed to need these foods, and you ignore nature at your peril. You can eat fruit and vegetables all day and you will not gain weight. We call the plant compounds that we identify as potentially important to us phytochemicals, which simply means plant-derived chemicals. The term *phytochemical* applies to fruits, vegetables, herbs, spices, and medicinal plants.

Eat your vegetables, even if you don't like them much. Consider that if you want to get in better shape and lose fat, your options are (1) to eat even smaller portions of foods that you like or (2) to eat the same portions and many more (mostly non-starchy) vegetables. Even if this is the lesser of two evils, most dieters don't want to eat even less than they already have to.

If you like fruit better than vegetables, eat more fruit, but remember that fruits always count as carbohydrate calories. Some diabetics cannot eat more than four pieces of fruit per day, so start with four as an upper limit. After you have improved your blood sugar control, you may increase your intake. However, produce of any kind is better than sugar or flour. Try to always eat your fruit raw. Check out a variety of fruits, especially tropical fruits such as mangoes, papayas, bananas, or Asian pears. Eat the peels whenever appropriate. Raw fruits also provide you with many important nutrients. Fruit juices are *not* a substitute for fruit, unless they are homemade with a whole fruit juice machine such as a Vita-Mix.

The same principle applies to vegetables—raw is best. Eating a small raw spinach salad, for example, is as good as a huge bowl of cooked spinach. If there is something you prefer, such as carrots, eat them raw every day. Make salads at home from scratch. Coleslaw is super-healthful, but not the nasty high-fat, low-flavor supermarket or deli stuff. Use a food processor and shred your own cabbage, carrots, and so forth and put on your own dressing. You can put anything in coleslaw from jalapeños to dill pickles to cold cooked chopped broccoli. Eat raw vegetables and dip for dinner. Eat lots of salsa, if you like it. Buy fresh, ripe produce, whether from farmers' markets or from your own garden. Get in the habit of slicing fresh home grown tomatoes on your dinner plate, for example, and eating them bite for bite with your meat or fish.

It's far better to eat starchy vegetables than to consume

starches in other forms, such as pasta, bread, or rice, although such vegetables do need to be counted as carbohydrate calories. Even though a potato, for example, does have a significant amount of carbohydrates, unless it's a potato chip, it's still mostly water. Not many people will eat three plain baked potatoes at one sitting, but three rolls are no problem. Corn, white and sweet potatoes, winter squash, beets, peas, jicama, yucca, and fresh (nondry) beans such as lima, shelly, and fava are all starchy vegetables. Unfortunately, people usually do not find starchy vegetables as tasty as pasta, bread, and rice. If this is true for you, try to eat the starchy vegetables instead of these other foods whenever you can, easing yourself into the Modern Evolutionary Diet. Keep in mind that eating these vegetables in place of carbohydrates in the form of sugars, rice, bread, and pasta *helps* you lose fat. Start to think of the bread, pasta, or rice that you love as a treat or dessert, not as a main course in your diet.

Green Power Foods

Green power food means a little snack of vegetables to get us back into our healthful evolutionary mode. It is best if this snack is raw, but it doesn't have to be. The snack can be carrot or celery sticks, a tomato or cucumber, a little leftover vegetable from another meal, or some salsa on cabbage or lettuce leaves. If you are on the run, try one of the various green drinks on the market, or spirulina, chlorella, or wheat or barley grass tablets. Start off with a little and increase as you go. If you cannot eat raw foods for one reason or another, you can buy small cans (or even baby food jars) of vegetables. Microwave squash for a snack, instead of popcorn or pastries. Get yourself in the habit of eating more vegetables, more often, and appreciate them for what they are and the great health benefits they give us. This is also the only way you can set a good example for your children.

Green Drinks

Green drinks are a special type of green power food chock-full of phytochemicals. Most green drinks combine various fruit, vegetable, seaweed, and herbal extracts. Green drinks also provide absorbable vitamins and minerals and often contain active enzymes and probiotics. They are like a large salad in a glass and are a natural appetite suppressant.

Green drinks are usually dark green coarse powders that are designed to be mixed in a beverage. They cost more than preparing your own salads, but are a convenient and painless way to add vegetable servings to your diet. They are an excellent way to start, if you don't like vegetables or are not currently eating very many and not enthusiastic about changing this policy. Green drinks can be mixed with any cold beverage. They can also be added to blender drinks, milk, yogurt, soft tofu, kefir, cottage cheese, fruit salad, or applesauce. Use green drinks with water as a green power food, or mixed with anything you like as a snack, along with a little protein.

Pollen

Bee pollen is the king of green power foods. It consists of blended pollen grains collected by honeybees from a wide variety of plants. Pollen is a major food source for the bees, and worker bees travel from flower to flower, collecting pollen in special "baskets" on their legs. Workers collect more than the hive needs, and beekeepers devise screens to scrape off some pollen as the bees enter the hive. Pollen, the male reproductive part of plants, is a very concentrated source of nutrients.

- Pollen contains every vitamin known, although B_{12} is low.
- Pollen is up to 40 percent protein, with a complete spectrum of amino acids.
- Over 25 trace elements account for 3.8 weight percent of pollen, including every essential trace element.

- Pollen contains 2–3 grams of fat per ounce. Most of the fats are PUFA: 70 percent alpha-linolenic (n-3), 3–4 percent linoleic (n-6), and 16–17 percent monounsaturated and saturated.
- Pollen contains numerous active enzymes and coenzymes.
- Pollen is uniformly rich in the beneficial phytochemicals called carotenoids, bioflavonoids, and phytosterols, but the exact profile is variable depending on the plant sources and growing conditions. However, beta-carotene, lycopene, beta-sitosterol, quercetin, isorhamnetin, kaempferol, and rutin have always been present in analyses of bee pollen.

Just like the green drinks, bee pollen is a superior and painless way to add servings of produce to your diet. Two teaspoons of bee pollen is the equivalent of a hearty serving of vegetables. Purchase pollen only in fresh, soft granules, and at first take only a few granules, to make sure you are not allergic to it (rare in healthy persons, but it does occur), and increase to up to a tablespoon at once. Fresh pollen is soft and pliable, smells flowery (like raw honey), and has not been heat treated. Good manufacturers gently double-crack pollen grains to ensure that the pollen is digestible.

Physically chewing the pollen is best for dieting. However, if you can't get used to the taste, mix or chase it with other food and swallow whole, or order bee pollen granules that have been encapsulated. Bee pollen is always blended from many different gatherings, and needs to be considered as a fresh produce-type food. Therefore, just like fresh fruits and vegetables, pollen is intrinsically variable, perishable, and subject to mishandling. If you happen to be allergic at first or don't like the quality of a product, don't give up—just send it back with a letter indicating that you wish to try a different lot number. Bee pollen greatly helps recovery from illness and injury and is also helpful for prostate inflammation.

Saying That We Should Eat No More Meat Is People Abuse

"The most damaging concept to our health today is that we would all be better off if we were vegetarians," nutritionist and author Robert Crayhon said to me. "And with this idea usually comes the assertion that humans are somehow 'designed' to be vegetarians. All of this is fallacious. If we are designed to eat anything, it is to eat animal products and uncultivated fruits and vegetables. For the vast majority of our history, we never ate grains, and the recent introduction (around 10,000 years ago) of grain products has caused more problems than it has solved. Before grains, diseases such as hypertension, heart disease, and diabetes were rare or unknown.

"You can eat a vegetarian diet and be healthy. It can be done. And there are those who seem to do all right on more carbohydrates and grains. It is just a lot harder to achieve optimal health as a vegetarian. You are more likely to be pulled down the path of too many carbohydrates and inadequate protein. Worst of all, you are eating a diet that your body was not designed for. You are an omnivore, no matter what your favorite columnist in your health magazine tells you. Limiting yourself to one part of the food spectrum limits your health.

"The criticisms one hears of meat-based diets are correct," Crayhon continued. "We need to increase the quality of animal products and stop animal abuse. We need to increase the quality of our animal products by not drugging animals with antibiotics and hormones. We need to feed animals grasses, flaxseeds, and other things that will increase the n-3 PUFA content of meat and other animal products. But saying that we should eat no meat is wrong. It is people abuse. It weakens our health and denies us the diet we were designed to eat: one which features meat as well as vegetables.

"A healthy vegetarian diet is far better than the junk-food-laden standard American fare. But it still pales in comparison to the health-promoting power of a diet built on Paleolithic principles. If the diet on which we developed contained animal products, and our development as humans depended on them, it is illogical to conclude that an optimal diet must now suddenly exclude them.

"Vegetarianism's benefits are the benefits of getting half of the Paleolithic picture right: eating lots of vegetables, as well as avoiding junky meat products. Evidence shows that vegetarians get more antioxidants like vitamin C and carotenoids through their diet, and this is good. But eating more vegetables is not something only vegetarians can do," Crayhon said. "Meat eaters should as well, while also moving toward more health-promoting fresh meat products. Vegetarians, through their blanket condemnation of meat, are in essence practicing foodism: they reject it all because some of it—bologna, high-fat meats, and aged meat—is health impairing.

"But the benefits of eating a lot of vegetables would only be furthered if the other half of the Paleolithic picture were added: the inclusion of high-quality, antibiotic- and hormone-free animal products from free-range animals or the nearest equivalent."

Breakfast

Eat mostly ripe, raw fruit and plain protein for breakfast. Take advantage of the season and farmers' markets if you can. Make a blender drink, try a fruit salad, or simply eat fruit whole. Eat as much as you desire—you can consume it over the course of several hours, if you want. Cooked or canned fruits are not allowed; frozen and thawed are all right sometimes, such as one component of a fruit salad. Some of the best fruits are melons, bananas, apricots, mangoes, peaches, pears, apples, kiwi, and red or black grapes—but seasonal fruits should take priority. Plain protein means two eggs and three egg whites cooked together, protein powder, turkey, chicken, cottage cheese, plain yogurt, low-fat sausage or hot dogs, or tuna fish. If you make no real distinction for breakfast-type foods, you'll do fine. If you can't stomach tuna fish in the morning, try plain yogurt or cottage cheese with a scoop of protein powder, your own fruit added, and a few chopped nuts sprinkled on top.

Late Morning

If you become hungry long before lunch, drink a green power food with 8 ounces skim or 2 percent milk, yogurt, soy milk, or water. Add some flax meal, if you like. If you use water, add a little protein food such as several egg whites, a piece of jerky, or a few nuts. You can also eat 1–3 teaspoons of bee pollen. If you don't need to eat, save these things for lunch.

Lunch

Have a green power food mixed with milk, cottage cheese, or yogurt and bee pollen if you did not have it already. You can also mix a green power food with water and eat any type of lean protein along with it. Otherwise, eat a large serving of protein of any type, fruit, and vegetables. Eat as many fresh vegetables as you can, preferably raw. Minimize the use of canned or frozen produce. High consumption of garlic, onion, peppers of all types, cabbage, carrots, beets, parsnips, turnips, broccoli, tomatoes, watercress, sprouts, and leafy green vegetables is encouraged. Blender drinks are great also. Have a high-protein sports nutrition bar for a treat or dessert, if you like.

Midafternoon

Same as late morning, if you are hungry long before dinner.

Dinner

Just before dinner, eat your green power food, if you did not have it in the afternoon. Eat fish, skinless poultry, or lean meat, homemade coleslaw, spinach salad, or sliced home-grown tomatoes with onions, and oven-roasted potatoes, lima beans, or corn. Make your own or use nonfat or low-fat salad dressings—there are many options now available. Eat all the vegetables you want—stuff yourself—but don't cover vegeta-bles with oily dressings and butter. Blender drinks are great for dinner also.

Dinner is the meal most likely to cause conflicts with your new diet, because it's the meal most likely shared with family or friends. Dishes based on pasta and macaroni are out, but you can make a lasagna, for example, with low-fat or fat-free ricotta cheese, browned 90 percent lean (or better) ground beef, turkey, or chicken, and half the noodles you would usu-ally use. Use slices of parcooked zucchini, eggplant, or yellow squash for half the noodle layers. If you make a spicy, garlicky sauce, and use plenty of meat and cheese (albeit lean ver-sions), you will have absolutely no complaints worth listening to.

Chinese, Korean, Indian, Japanese, and similar Asian cuisines food are simply eaten without rice and bread. Order mainly sashimi instead of sushi when eating Japanese, and skip the lo mein and dan-dan noodles when eating Chinese. Have soup or steamed meat dumplings for an appetizer. Don't order deep-fried dishes or appetizers, or any dish with an excessively sweet sauce.

Skip the greasy deep-fried appetizers, samosas, rice biryani, and breads when eating Indian foods. Order or cook a tan-doori dish or a vindaloo, and ask for a sampler of fresh salads and chutneys. If you love the delicious Indian naan bread as much as I do, have one, but stick to tandoori shrimp or chicken as a meal. Alternatively, get one to go and eat it later for dessert. You can lose fat faster if you can eat only shrimp and salad, but we all don't have such discipline. What I'm try-ing to get you to avoid is the Indian cuisine standard practice of covering a big dish of rice with very greasy lamb (or vegetarian!) curry sauce. If you make these choices firmly, quietly, and politely, nobody need even know that you are on a diet. You will avoid any unnecessary talk about your situation, and without even trying, you can set a good eating example for others.

Generally avoid one-pot dishes such as paella, couscous, casseroles, and noodle soups. Instead, pick dishes in which you can keep your protein separate, and dishes that are not based on grains. Evaluate common foods by using the guidelines; for example, chili with lots of lean meat, onions, tomatoes, peppers, and a few beans is a much better choice than high-fat, high-carbohydrate macaroni and cheese. Chili is also a better choice than a typical Vietnamese noodle soup (Pho), which is lower in fat but packed with noodles and garnished with only a few slices of meat. You would have to eat many bowls of the macaroni and cheese or soup to get the protein you need, but one bowl of chili suffices. Although I have cautioned you about beans, we are using beans for the carbohydrate source in this chili meal, not the protein source.

In short, you can make any meal work for you and most (if not all) family members by getting the idea out of your head that you are going to use some sort of grain or bean combining to get balanced protein. If you try to do this, as both a diabetic and a dieter, your intake of carbohydrates will be unacceptably high, meal after meal. This type of eating strategy is for a person who has absolutely no need to restrict calories or carbohydrates. Furthermore, grain or bean combining was not the nutritional strategy that we evolved eating. It is a strategy based on subsistence agriculture, and we have already established that humans evolved in the absence of agriculture.

Snacks, Desserts, Light Meals, and Treats

Try to stay off these altogether, or at least until you have lost one-third to one-half of the weight you wish to. But just in case, here are some alternatives. Nobody is a dietary saint, and once in a while we like a treat or something sweet. Many of these suggestions are good ideas for healthful children's snacks also. Please try to avoid the new wave of fat-free and low-fat commercial baked goods. They are mainly just junk food minus some of the hydrogenated fat. It is very hard to stop eating low-fat cookies and pastries once you start. Instead, try one of the following.

High-protein sports nutrition bars
Bee pollen snack bars
Low-fat granola or fig bars
Cafe latte, mocha, cappuccino, etc. (get the regular type, not nonfat)
Hot chocolate or chocolate milk
Banana spread with nut butter
One serving of bread, cereal, or granola of any type (you can have bread spread with nut butter)
Cooked or canned fruit with a little cream
Cashews, peanuts, pecans, or other slightly sweet nuts
Trail mix
Commercial fruit-flavored yogurt
Sugar-free pudding

What If I'm Hungry Between or Right Before Meals?

If you find that hunger pangs regularly make it impossible to wait until mealtimes, you could try one or more of the following strategies.

1. Keep preservative-free meat and fish jerkies or low-fat meat sticks around. A little goes a long way to stop hunger pangs. Eat some jerky with an apple, pear, or other crunchy raw fruit—and take a few minutes to chew and swallow.
2. Keep hard-boiled eggs in your home or workplace refrigerator. Eat only the whites as snacks or as protein added

to a salad or other foods with meals. Egg whites are amazing in their ability to act as appetite suppressants.

3. Eat some bee pollen with a huge glass of water.
4. Hot drinks are effective at suppressing appetite, especially coffee and some of the herbal teas. Try half coffee and half sugar-free hot chocolate, and use a little cream. A little cream and no sugar will keep your stomach quieter than no cream and a lot of sugar. The fat in a single-serving container of half-and-half is not really significant.
5. Increase the fiber content of your diet. Eat more vegetables, and try drinking 2–3 teaspoons of flax meal mixed in a full glass of water before meals. Flax meal is made from food-grade flaxseed with the flaxseed oil pressed out. Also try mixing flax meal with a green drink. Flax meal provides an extremely high amount of fiber, prevents constipation, suppresses appetite, and helps normalize blood sugar. It also supplies potassium, zinc, B vitamins, PUFA, and trace elements. It is the world's highest food source of lignans, which can help prevent reproductive cancers. Flax meal can be mixed in any beverage or blender drink, used in baking, or cooked with hot cereals. It can even be cooked in the microwave with only water. Start with 1–1½ teaspoons twice per day and increase to 2–3 teaspoons twice per day.
6. Try high-protein sports nutrition bars. Some of my favorites are named in the Resources section or you can find at least a dozen bar selections in any health food store. Read the labels, and look for one with over 12 grams of protein per 200 to 300 calories of bar. Ignore the fat content—pick what you like.

8

Supplements, Sweeteners, and Maintaining or Gaining Weight

The basic supplement plan is critical to the success of the Modern Evolutionary Diet and essential for preventing or reversing diabetes. Other chapters have more suggestions for herbs and specialty supplements to help control blood sugar and improve diabetic complications, and these additional supplements are intended to work with the basic plan, not replace it. All nutrients are synergistic. In this chapter, there is also a piggy-back supplement plan for aiding fat loss. All supplements should be taken with meals or snacks, unless otherwise noted. Suggestions for actual products are given in the Resources section.

Modern Evolutionary Diet Basic Supplement Plan

Morning Supplements

1 multivitamin/multimineral

Make sure that the one you take has at least 30 mg of vitamin B complex and 15–25 mg of zinc in the suggested total daily dosage. Note that your choice may require 1, 2, 3, or more capsules or tablets per day. Pick a supplement that fits with your lifestyle—if you can't remember to take 3 capsules per day, don't choose that supplement.

Supermarket multivitamins with RDA levels of nutrients are not sufficient.

1 balanced antioxidant supplement

Make sure that the one you take has a total of 400 IU of vitamin E and 50–200 mcg of selenium in the total suggested daily dosage. Choose one that has both antioxidant vitamins and botanical products. Note that your choice may require more than 1, 2, 3, or more capsules or tablets per day. Again, pick a supplement that fits with your lifestyle. Supermarket antioxidants with RDA levels of nutrients are not sufficient.

500–1,000 mg vitamin C with bioflavonoids
200–400 mg magnesium
250–500 mg calcium (Do not use calcium carbonate or
    calcium oxide.)
1–2 teaspoons flaxseed or Essential Balance oil (If you weigh
    over 170 pounds, take 2 teaspoons.)

Note: If you don't like to eat breakfast, have a green drink and some bee pollen with your supplements.

Midmorning Supplements

Green power food, if you didn't have any in the morning. Use with a protein food, if you're eating a snack.

Midday Supplements

2,000 mg fish oil
2,000 mg evening primrose oil

Note: Avoid carbonated beverages when taking the oil capsules. If oil capsules bother you, take them on an empty stomach before or a few hours after midday.

200 mcg chromium picolinate
500–1,000 mg vitamin C with bioflavonoids
1 multivitamin/multimineral, if the one you choose has three divided doses
1 balanced antioxidant supplement, if the one you choose has three divided doses

Midafternoon Supplements (or Before Dinner on an Empty Stomach)

Green power food

Use with a protein food if you're eating a snack.

Evening Supplements

1–2 teaspoons flaxseed or Essential Balance oil (If you weigh over 170 pounds, take 2 teaspoons.)
1 multivitamin/multimineral, if the one you choose has two or three divided doses
1 balanced antioxidant supplement, if the one you choose has two or three divided doses
500–1,000 mg vitamin C with bioflavonoids
200–400 mg magnesium
250–500 mg calcium

Do not use calcium carbonate or calcium oxide. If you consume very little calcium in your diet or are a pregnant, nursing, or postmenopausal woman, you need to take 800 to 1,000 mg of calcium total per day. On the other hand, if you are male and enjoy dairy products, you may need only 200 to 300 mg of calcium. You'll have to evaluate your own calcium consumption and needs. If you get a lot of calcium in your diet, 250 to 500 mg per day supplementation is sufficient.

200 mcg chromium picolinate

Note: If you are presently diabetic, you will need to take another 2,000 mg of fish oil and 2,000 mg of evening primrose oil. You will also need to take more chromium picoli-nate, but read Chapter 4 to determine how to safely phase in higher chromium doses. Magnesium and zinc supple-mentation may also need adjustments in a similar fashion (Chapter 4).

Piggy-Back Supplement Plan for Fat Loss

These additional supplements all have some scientific research backing up the claims that they can aid in body fat loss or improve body composition—that is, they can help us retain or gain lean tissue while losing fat. They are also com-pletely safe and nonstimulant, and so are not contraindicated for any health conditions or medications.

Take the following supplement on an empty stomach, morning or afternoon:

3,000 mg L-carnitine

Take the following supplements each morning, midday, and evening:

1–2 weight-loss blend with Citrin (tablets or capsules)

This may have Citrin (*Garcinia cambogia* herbal extract) only or may be a combined herbal supplement, and may also contain chromium picolinate. If so, adjust your chromium supplementation accordingly. Follow the manufacturer's recommendations for the number of pills to take at your weight.

4 capsules of HMB (beta-hydroxy methyl butyrate) (You need a total of 12 per day, so don't skimp here.)
1,000 mg CLA (conjugated linoleic acid)
2,000–3,000 mg potassium pyruvate

Don't skimp on these last two supplements either. Don't bother to take them if you're not willing to take the full dose. These are high-dose supplements.

Iron

This supplement plan may or may not be iron-free, based on your choice of multivitamin. Iron does not need to be supplemented beyond RDA levels (or at all), unless you have tested anemic. Most men do not need iron, and may even be harmed by excess iron—this is particularly true for diabetics. If you are or have been a vegetarian, especially one who consumes a lot of soy products, or are a premenopausal woman, you might need iron. Check with your doctor. If extra iron is needed, choose a 25 mg chelated iron supplement and take it every other day, separate from other supplements. It would be excellent to take it along with a green power food. Don't use ferrous sulfate. Levels of iron supplementation beyond about 25 mg per day are unnecessary, except in rare medical conditions, and cause nausea and constipation. Anemia in a relatively healthy person that does not respond to iron supplementation at this level is usually due to other existing nutrient imbalances or deficiencies, and a fully balanced supplement plan and a dietary evaluation should be done before iron supplementation is increased. Keep in mind that meat and seafood provide the most absorbable sources not only of iron, but also zinc, copper, and manganese. No other mineral supplements are utilized as well as these food sources—so those who eat a variety of meats and seafoods daily rarely have deficiencies of these trace elements.

Chromium

Chromium is lacking in virtually every diet. Since it is rarely added to multivitamins in a realistic dosage, we need to add it as an independent supplement. This trace element is an insulin cofactor—it is required for normal insulin function and glucose metabolism. Chapter 4 describes the importance of chromium in treating diabetes. Chromium picolinate has been shown to help humans build muscle, while losing fat. Chromium also lowers total blood cholesterol levels, by lowering LDL and raising HDL.

Vitamin C

Vitamin C is critical to every aspect of health. Always take at least 1,000 mg per day, even when you travel. This is perhaps the single most important vitamin to supplement at levels far in excess of the 60 mg RDA. Children need 500–1,000 mg per day also. Bioflavonoids are phytochemicals that are naturally found together with vitamin C in fruits and vegetables. Vitamin C is synergistic with bioflavonoids, and a good argument can be made that they should not be separated. Therefore choosing a vitamin C plus bioflavonoids supplement is recommended.

Flaxseed Oil

Flaxseed oil or Essential Balance oil (a flax oil blend) may be mixed in cold foods such as dips, cottage cheese, or salad dressings, used as a butter replacement on prepared foods, or taken by the spoon. They should never be used for cooking. Flaxseed oil and Essential Balance oil are nearly interchangeable and can be alternated for taste. Essential Balance Jr. is also available with a butterscotch flavor. Always purchase flax oil or flax oil blends in sealed black plastic bottles that have been refrigerated in the store. Flaxseed oil needs to be cold pressed, unrefined, and protected from heat and light. Your oil should have a pressing date and an expiration date on the label, and these dates need to be taken seriously. Inform the store if they are selling oil that will soon be or is already out of date. *Always* store these oils in the refrigerator. If you can't use up the oil fast enough, you can freeze it for longer storage.

Noncaloric Sweeteners

In making blender drinks, I often find that they are not sweet enough to suit my taste. I don't wish to add a lot of extra calories or sugar, so I add a tiny bit of stevia, trutina, or saccharin. These have no distinct taste when blended in with all the fruit and other ingredients, and act to balance the flavor.

Trutina and stevia are by far the best choices, but have been unavailable until recently and are still quite expensive. White stevia powder is a 100 percent natural, safe, concentrated, and calorie-free sweetener. It comes from the leaves of a type of chrysanthemum native to Paraguay. Stevia is great for sweetening tea, coffee, yogurt, or balancing blender drinks when fruit is too sour or not fully ripe. You can mix stevia with other sweeteners to help you reduce your sugar intake. Trutina comes from kiwi fruit, and is used similarly, but does cake up or clump if not sealed tightly.

Saccharin is a better choice than aspartame. Saccharin has been used for hundreds of years, with very few adverse affects reported in humans. Research indicating that saccharin is carcinogenic was performed by feeding test animals relative quantities of saccharin far in excess of what any human would eat in a lifetime. Furthermore, saccharin is restricted to individual packets and boxes and a few specialty products such as sugar-free tonic water. It is difficult to abuse saccharin when it is marketed in this fashion. Saccharin, cyclamates, and Acesulfame-K (the latter two are not generally available in the United States) are excreted unchanged by the kidneys. They are also stable in hot beverages and for long-term storage.

In contrast, aspartame is broken down to its constituent amino acids in the intestine (hence the phenylalanine warning on the label). It is not stable in warm or hot conditions, or during long-term storage. Heat decomposes this product into some distasteful and toxic compounds. Aspartame has found its way into breath mints, chewing gums, virtually all diet sodas, and thousands of foods. It has received more FDA consumer complaints than any other single product. Almost everyone has a friend or relative who is a diet soda addict. Under current market circumstances, the potential to abuse aspartame by consuming huge amounts is very real.

It's the dose that makes the poison. If you eat a sound Modern Evolutionary Diet, small amounts of any junk or artificial foods are not going to significantly harm you. Your body will be strong enough to detoxify them, if they are toxic. However, once these small amounts become large enough to crowd out "real" food, you are on your way to a self-destructive diet.

Maintaining Weight

If you are healthy and at normal weight, or have finished losing fat, here are some suggestions to continue eating healthful indefinitely. Following the Modern Evolutionary Diet is good insurance against future excess body fat gain due to aging, pregnancy, shifting to a sedentary job, or changing exercise habits.

1. Follow the diet but don't make a real effort to control portions.
2. Follow the diet 5 days per week and eat or drink whatever you like 2 days per week. If pounds sneak on, you know exactly why and exactly where to cut back.
3. About 20–25 percent of the diet calories may be from fat, as long as you first make sure you get your PUFA each day. Use low-fat or reduced-fat dairy and soy products instead of fat-free. Add more coconut oil, nut butters, and nut flours to blender drinks. Cook two eggs and two whites instead of all whites. You do not need to count the PUFA supplements or oils as fat calories.
4. Snack more liberally, using lean protein sources, snack bars, sports nutrition bars, nuts, and trail mix.
5. Discontinue specific weight loss supplements, but don't discontinue chromium supplementation.
6. Add prudent servings of cooked dried beans, whole grain breads and cereals, and other dried grain products to meals. *Add* is the operative word here. Do not start

replacing your meals and snacks with large servings of these foods, or you will be right back where you started. Think of them as side dishes to fill out an already balanced Evolutionary Diet meal.

7. No healthful diet includes large amounts of sugar, refined grains, sodas, candy, sweet baked goods, snack chips, or alcohol. If you must eat these foods at times, add them to the Modern Evolutionary Diet framework and consider them as nothing other than a source of calories to prevent actual weight loss. Realize that eating these foods deprives you of nutrients, rather than providing them.

Gaining Weight and Diets for Growing Children

By gaining weight, I mean gaining lean body mass rather than fat. If fat reserves are indeed extremely low, the body will normally correct this problem itself in any balanced, nutritionally sound weight gain program. However, it is impossible to gain muscle and bone mass without adequate protein, vitamins, and trace elements. Proper PUFA nutrition is also crucial for weight gain and growth, because PUFA are part of every cell membrane. In order to gain weight, your body must create or expand healthy cells at a relatively rapid rate. This means that your body needs access to good-quality raw materials at all times, and the Modern Evolutionary Diet is your best choice to provide those raw materials. After all, it's the diet that made it possible for your ancestors to cause *you* to be alive today!

Starting kids off on the Modern Evolutionary Diet when young helps ensure that they get the nutrients they need and teaches them good eating habits for life. Certainly children have a better attention span and do better in school if they eat balanced meals. High-carbohydrate diets, and meals and snack foods consisting mainly of processed carbohydrate and fat (like most junk food), are really tough on growing children. These foods set the stage for behavior problems, illness, and later eating disorders. After they have eaten a good meal, there are plenty of healthy treat snacks on the market to reward your kids with. Don't underestimate how much they will go for power blender drinks and power sports bars. Nuts, sports nutrition bars, trail mix, fruit spread with nut butter, and sweetened yogurt mixed with a little protein powder make good snacks for children.

Eight Suggestions for Weight Gain

As I said before, the weight gained is lean body mass, not fat.

1. Eat 3 "major" meals and 2 or 3 "minor" meals per day. Use blender drinks or sports nutrition bars for minor meals or *in addition* to meals, not *in place of* meals.
2. Calculate your daily protein requirement based on the lean body mass that you would like to achieve, instead of your present weight. Also use 1.0 for your activity factor. Avoid eating a lot of soy products and don't use soy protein powder, unless you must do so for allergy reasons. I recommend using cold-processed ion-exchanged whey protein powder daily for best results. If you are primarily weight training, continue to scale up your protein as you gain, and add carbs as appropriate for your duration and intensity of training.
3. Weight gain diets may be 20–30 percent fat. Young children should not have less than 30 percent fat and should never be given fat-free dairy products. They need the fat-soluble vitamins and the energy. You can make relatively liberal use of unrefined oils and nut butters; add quite a bit of coconut oil to blender drinks, and spread nut butters on fruits and vegetables. Use reduced-fat or whole dairy products and salad dressings. Add avocados, nuts, and grated hard cheese to salads. Eat a mix of whole eggs and egg whites. Eat a variety of fresh meats and seafood, but stick to leaner choices as a general rule. Eating low-fat protein most days of the week and splurging on prime

rib one day is better than eating a little too much animal fat every day. You do not need to count any PUFA supplements as fat calories.

4. Pay fairly strict attention to your protein/carbohydrate/fat ratio. The ideal ranges for persons trying to gain muscle are 20–30 percent of calories from fat, 30–40 percent from protein, and 30–50 percent from carbohydrate. No need to count carbs strictly, unless they come from grains, sugars, or beans. Eating protein throughout the day gives good results. Always eat a very high protein meal or snack right before bed, such as whey protein.

5. Eat high-protein sports nutrition bars, dried or fresh fruit, fruit, nuts, nut butters, and other healthful snack foods regularly.

6. You can use prudent amounts of royal jelly honey or other raw honey, fruit preserves and juices, or molasses instead of, or in addition to, noncaloric sweeteners. Fruit juices may be *added* to meals but not used in place of fresh fruit. Eat larger servings of potatoes, sweet potatoes, lima beans, and corn. Cooked, canned, and dried fruits may be consumed.

7. Pasta, breads, cereals, cooked beans and grains, and reasonable desserts may be added to an evolutionary meal framework of lean protein and fresh vegetables, but not used in place of it. Weight lifting or other athletic training is certainly not enhanced in the long run by consuming excessive amounts of carbohydrate. Increasing your total calories, while keeping your protein, fat, and carbohydrate relatively balanced, provides you with abundant energy. Keep in mind that the Modern Evolutionary Diet does not bother to count the carbohydrates found in most vegetables. If you do strenuous aerobic athletic training, use the Modern Evolutionary Diet as a base for your first 2,000 or so calories, and then add carbohydrates as needed for performance energy. However, if you want to be healthy and diabetes-free,

avoid basing meals on dried grain agricultural products as much as possible.

8. A need or desire to gain weight is not a license to eat whatever you want. On the contrary, it is an incentive to provide yourself with only the best-quality food, especially protein of high biological value. You are trying to recreate your body! Dried grain agricultural products are inferior sources of energy and nutrients. The more refined they are, the worse they are. No healthful diet includes large amounts of sugar, refined grains, sodas, candy, sweet baked goods, snack chips, or alcohol. You cannot grow muscle with sugar and flour, no matter how hard you try.

9

Putting the Modern Evolutionary Diet into Practice

In terms of meal planning, "Keep it simple" is our motto. If you can't clearly identify which foods contain mostly protein, carbohydrate, or fat, or can't separate the carbohydrate components of your foods from the protein and fat components (as in pancakes or casseroles), you are working too hard. In general, meals consist of plain lean protein, two to four vegetables (or a mix of fruits and vegetables), and a little fat. Foods made from dried grains, beans, flour, or sugar are excluded. The fat can be from a variety of unprocessed sources, and needs to contain balanced PUFA on average for the day or over the course of several days. Fats may come from salad dressings, nuts, avocados, egg yolks, meat, fish, coconut oil or other oils in the blender drink recipe, or some butter-fat from dairy products. Fried foods, junk foods with hydrogenated fats, and high-fat meats and cheeses are excluded.

This means that chef salads take the place of sandwiches in your life. Pizza and pasta are out. Save them for your day off the diet, if you must. Raw vegetables in dips replace chips. Skip bread, noodles, and rice side dishes. Don't waste your time or your tooth enamel learning to cook whole grains—your family won't eat them anyway. Breakfasts are high-protein meals, not oversized bagels, doughnuts, or muffins.

Power blender drinks are a fundamental part of putting the

Modern Evolutionary Diet into practice, and a master recipe and example flavors are given below. Blender drinks help you increase the amount of high-quality protein in your diet effortlessly, and are always available to save you, if your sweet tooth threatens to get the better of you. Keep in mind, though, that once you get adequate PUFA, protein, vitamins, and trace elements in your body for a few weeks, and address any food allergies you might have, a lot of food you craved and thought you could never live without will become relatively unimportant. Many diets recommend eating five or six small snack-like meals throughout the day instead of fewer, larger meals. This is good advice for keeping up energy levels, and may tend to keep your metabolic rate a bit higher and reduce the tendency to store fat. However, it is not a plan that works for everyone. It may be impossible for you to do, if your job or schedule does not permit this type of eating. Even worse, it is not a good option for those who have difficulty stopping eating once they start. It can lead to repeated defeats, when you blow your diet by consuming too many calories early in the day, and then just give up and keep on overeating for the remainder of the day. If you have difficulty stopping eating once you start, plan your largest meal for dinner and eat heartily then. Eat very nutritiously and sparingly during the day, consuming mostly egg whites, other plain protein, fruits, vegetables, bee pollen, and other green power foods. Eat just to maintain your energy level, but do not starve yourself or fast. Plain protein is the best food for controlling hunger with a minimum of calories, and cooked egg whites in particular have an appetite-suppressant effect.

Meal Planning

For each meal, I have given a suggestion for every day of the week. It's a good idea to keep track of what works for you and what does not, and then make up your own 7-day list. Plan each week at a time for 2 months or so, and then without even thinking, you will be eating the Modern Evolutionary Diet way. Consult the Resources section for suggestions for particular

brand names and suppliers of some of the products mentioned here.

Breakfast

DAY 1. Plain yogurt, cottage cheese, or kefir with your own fresh
fruit added and a few chopped nuts sprinkled on top. Even better: swirl in a tablespoon of liquid protein, any flavor.

DAY 2. Blender drink of any flavor you like.

DAY 3. Two eggs and two egg whites cooked any style and served with salsa.

DAY 4. Two high-protein sports nutrition bars and two teaspoons of bee pollen.

DAY 5. Several slices lean turkey or chicken breast, cold cuts,
or a dish of cooked egg whites; raw carrots and celery; and a
sports nutrition bar.

DAY 6. A dish of cooked egg whites, several slices lean turkey,
chicken breast, or ham, and a fruit salad drizzled with
flaxseed or Essential Balance oil and sprinkled with flax meal.

DAY 7. Denver omelette with two eggs and two egg whites and
fresh fruit.

Lunch

DAY 1. BLT chef salad or spinach salad with turkey bacon, apple
cider or sherry vinegar, and garlic-chili flavored flaxseed oil.
You can use hard-cooked eggs (two eggs plus two whites) or
reduced-fat cheese instead of the bacon. Or treat yourself to
smoked salmon, sable, mackerel, or trout on the salad.

DAY 2. Sliced turkey breast and succotash.

DAY 3. Make yogurt or kefir cheese by straining kefir just like
yogurt. Commercial strainers are available or use a fine
sieve or coffee filter. Top baked potatoes with kefir cheese
and Essential Balance Jr. oil. Eat with a few slices of low-fat
ham or turkey.

DAY 4. Stir-fried tofu and mixed vegetables, or a light oriental
dish, but skip the rice and noodles. Or treat yourself to a
sashimi lunch.

DAY 5. Cottage cheese, yogurt, or kefir, with fruit, flax meal, and few chopped nuts, or some Essential Balance oil.

DAY 6. Cold smoked or poached fish, sliced tomatoes and cucumbers, sports nutrition bar or trail mix.

DAY 7. Blender drink.

Snack

DAY 1. Green power food and fruit.

DAY 2. Sports nutrition bar, bee pollen, and coffee.

DAY 3. 1–2 ounces of nuts and celery sticks.

DAY 4. Celery or carrots spread with nut butter.

DAY 5. Leftover cold chicken, turkey, fish, or shellfish with raw vegetables.

DAY 6. Hard-boiled egg whites, bee pollen, sports nutrition bar.

DAY 7. Mini-chef salad or leftover coleslaw with shrimp or tuna fish added.

Dinner

DAY 1. Grilled marinated skinless chicken breasts or thighs, roasted peppers, onions, and zucchini and/or yellow squash. Try curry-marinated or tandoori chicken for a spicy change.

DAY 2. Ostrich meat, which is a very lean red meat raised free-range that can be purchased by mail order or at specialty markets. Ostrich is similar to wild game, but has a milder flavor. Try a grilled or roasted ostrich tenderloin, with green salad and roasted potatoes. Substitute pork tenderloin, venison, or beef eye of round, very well trimmed. Use flaxseed oil dressing on the salad.

DAY 3. Peel and eat boiled spiced shrimp, corn on the cob, and coleslaw.

DAY 4. Make your favorite hunter's stew or Irish stew recipe with venison or turkey. Use two or three times the vegetables called for in the standard recipe. Or try your favorite seafood stew or jambalaya, but skip the rice and bread.

DAY 5. Baked skinless chicken breasts or salmon steaks, baked winter squash, and green beans. Use Essential Balance Jr. on the squash.

DAY 6. Blender drink, or cottage, kefir, or yogurt cheese with fruit and Essential Balance Jr.

DAY 7. Make your favorite spaghetti sauce. Use ground turkey, chicken, ostrich, venison, or 93 percent lean ground beef. Brown meat and drain off all fat. Or use lean turkey Italian sausage. Cook spaghetti squash, green beans, or zucchini and put the sauce on top. Do the same with chili, but skip the beans or use one can of black beans only in a whole recipe.

Note: If you stick closely to the Evolutionary Diet Plan, you may have any sports nutrition bar, granola bar, fig bars, or other healthful snack bar later on for "dessert." Fresh fruits with a little cream, sour cream, kefir, or yogurt, and a sprinkle of cinnamon is also a nice dessert. Add chocolate liquid protein—it tastes like Hershey's syrup! One serving of bread, dry cereal, trail mix, or a banana spread with nut butter are other options. Before having your treat, finish your meal, clean up the dishes, brush your teeth, and wait at least one hour.

Seven Things to Do When You're on the Go

1. In fast-food restaurants, choose a grilled or rotisserie chicken or roast beef sandwich. Discard the chicken skin or bun. Try the salad bar, fill up, and enjoy.
2. Take with you on the road: high-protein sports nutrition bars; fruit; beef, buffalo, fish, or turkey jerky; ostrich meat sticks; bee pollen; hard-boiled eggs; nuts; and green drinks. Stop in any convenience store for cold spring water. Power Bars and Balance Bars are also available in almost every large chain convenience store.
3. Ask the deli to put turkey, lettuce, tomatoes, pickles, onions, and so forth on a plate for you. Skip the sub roll and put some mustard, relish, and a *little* mayo on the side. Avoid pizza, doughnuts, muffins, and bagels.
4. Ask the oriental restaurant to go very light on the stir-fry

oil for you and send your food back if they don't. Choose light dishes (no deep-fried foods or sweet, heavy sauces) and skip the rice and noodles.

5. In a Mexican restaurant, ask for a taco salad without the taco shell or the cheese. Get double salsa and guacamole on top, and sour cream only if the fat-free kind is offered.

6. Measure out protein powder and carry it with you in a large plastic container. Purchase frozen or regular yogurt, as plain as possible. Mix yogurt into the protein powder. If you can get plain yogurt or cottage cheese while on the road, it's a good idea to mix in your own fruit, or a green drink powder, and even stevia or trutina to sweeten it gently.

7. Carry green drinks with you when you know you won't be able to get any fresh vegetables. Just mix them with water. You can also buy a small jar of mild salsa in any convenience store and eat the whole thing plain as a vegetable dish. One serving of any green power food, 2 teaspoons of bee pollen, or a half-serving green drink plus 2 teaspoons of flaxseed meal (for the fiber) each count as a generous serving of vegetables. Alternatively, pay extra at supermarket salad bars, if you don't have time to make salads. Your health is worth it, and besides, have you checked out the outrageous prices for repackaged flour, fat, salt, and sugar in the junk food aisles?

Kicking a Sugar or Starch Addiction

If you are a sugar or starch addict, and feel that there is *no way* you can stop eating these foods at every meal, don't despair but do follow my advice. First, get all the foods you cheat on *out of the house!* Tell yourself that if you want something terribly badly, you can have it, but you must go out to get it. This applies to family members also. If they complain that their favorite junk food is not around the house, tell them to go out for it themselves. If they are too young to go out, have an older member of the family help, or maybe they can just suffer. Have more healthful snacks or snacks that are *not* your favorites around the house instead.

Whenever you have cravings for sugar or starch, drink a large glass of cold water or plain tea with two tablespoons of raw apple cider vinegar or lemon juice. You can add a little noncaloric sweetener, if you wish, but no sugar. Also, slowly eat a little bit of plain protein, such as a few hard-boiled egg whites, plain chicken, or tuna. A little bee pollen helps greatly as well. Tell yourself that you have to wait only 15 minutes to eat sugar or starch. After 15 minutes, if the craving is still strong, do the same again with the acidified water and protein. Then busy yourself with something that needs to be done that you never seem to have the time to do, such as cleaning out a shelf, hand-washing a blouse, scrubbing out the trash can, or walking around the yard. If you still have a craving, eat the same thing you did earlier, and add some plain raw vegetables, if you wish. After 15 more minutes, you will be fine. If not, if you must go out to buy what you crave, do so—but you won't eat as much as you used to. For the first 2–4 days, all this will be difficult, no doubt, so don't even try to count calories—*just try to follow the plan.* Eat as much protein as you can handle. If you can successfully avoid the sugar siren song in this manner, you will diminish your cravings in a matter of days and your attempts at dieting may finally begin to show some success. If you have no success with this program and tend to have "hypoglycemia" and other health problems as well, you may have a systemic Candida yeast infection or food allergies. If this is the case, you need to consult Chapter 11.

What about sweetened sodas? Remove them from your diet. To wean yourself off soda, start by mixing ⅔ soda with ⅓ unsweetened soda water. The cherry-, lemon-, lime-, and raspberry-flavored soda waters are especially nice. Then move to 50/50 and eventually to ⅔ soda water and ⅓ soda. You can do it, just try, and don't spoil your palate by sipping the regular soda first! No stocking up at home by purchasing six-packs on sale either. Keep it away from your kids too—it makes them inattentive, sugar-addicted, hyperactive, and nutrient-deficient.

If you must, clandestinely mix fruit juice with soda water and put it inside empty orange or grape 2-liter soda bottles to fool young kids or give them diet soda only. If you crave soda, go to a convenience store and buy one soda for an exorbitant price. Then you will treat it with reverence. Always drink water first when you are thirsty, and then go on to something else, if you must.

Nutritionist Tells All

In explaining his clinical success with his version of the Modern Evolutionary Diet, nutritionist and author Robert Crayhon said, "I have found that returning to a diet that contains more animal protein (especially wild game) and less food of civilization (especially less grains and refined carbohydrates) to be one of the most valuable tools I use clinically to help people recover from a wide range of chronic illnesses. Most people feel better on less grain and more meat, and it makes sense—this is what we ate for the vast majority of our history as humans. I myself was a vegetarian for 11 years, but my health improved markedly after returning to meat and greatly reducing grain consumption.

"I work with a group of over 30 nutritionists in the New York metropolitan area, and we have found that excessive carbohydrate and inadequate protein consumption, combined with inadequate intake of essential fatty acids, to be the main dietary problems our clients have. Changing their diets to a more historically based one, higher in protein and lower in grains, alleviates food cravings and yeast overgrowths, and increases energy levels. Blood lipids improve, especially HDL cholesterol, which goes up. It may be that much of the heart disease we see is due to inadequate protein consumption, which leads to low levels of protective HDL."

What to Do If You Need to Cheat

Cheating is part of any diet. It is better to know your enemy and meet him face to face than wait for him to ambush you. If you understand and follow the Modern Evolutionary Diet fairly closely, you can allow yourself some latitude. It may mean that you do not lose fat as quickly, or that you do not perform at your absolute best, but you will still be far ahead of your junk food and carbohydrate addict peers.

1. Take one day off per week and eat whatever you want.
2. Eat oatmeal or another cooked hot cereal (no dry box cereals) in the morning, if you want to, but add some protein to the meal. Adding a scoop of protein powder to the hot cereal is a great way to do this.
3. Skip all carbs at dinner, but save that homemade bread for at least 1 hour after dinner and eat it as a dessert.
4. There are other options if you skip all carbs at a meal and want a treat later: 1–3 ounces of nuts or trail mix; gourmet coffee with a little cream or whole milk; mocha with half coffee and half sugar-free or reduced-sugar cocoa; raisin bran bagel or whole grain raisin toast with a little nut butter or soft cheese; oatmeal or whole grain breakfast cereal with milk; cottage cheese; a few nuts and dried fruits such as raisins or cherries.
5. If it's a party, choose your cheating wisely. A rack of BBQ ribs or a steak are better choices than a bowl of corn or potato chips or a rich dessert. You won't want to eat ribs again the next day, but you will certainly crave the chips and cake!
6. If you plan to drink alcohol at a social occasion, drink away, but eat only protein and nonstarchy vegetables. In other words, take your carbs in the form of beer or wine. Drink 12–16 ounces of plain water for every alcoholic beverage you consume. Avoid drinking liquor mixed with soda, but fruit or tomato juices are all right. Drink 16 ounces of cold water and take a multivitamin, 1,000

mg of vitamin C, and two capsules of milk thistle herb before you go to bed.

7. If you must snack, eat protein or bee pollen and drink water first. Then do the same again. Then eat sports nutrition bars next. Nuts are a good choice, also. Eating the right food here is more important than counting calories, but if you snack a lot on anything, you will not lose weight. However, if you keep this snack plan in mind, you may not overeat in your snacking. If you immediately give in and start eating serious junk when you snack, you will overeat in your snacking every time.

8. If you can't quit chocolate, don't! Just stay away from cheap, junk food sugar- and preservative-laden chocolate. Also avoid anything made with chocolate and wheat, such as cakes, cookies, and doughnuts. For those devoted to chocolate, four strategies follow.

a. Eat chocolate sports nutrition bars for any snack or meal.

b. Make chocolate blender drinks.

c. Drink coffee mixed with sugar-free hot chocolate or hot chocolate alone, using a bit of cream, of course. Make homemade chocolate pudding. Eat a plain green salad and chocolate pudding, with a scoop or two of protein powder, for lunch every single day, if you need to. Do whatever it takes to avoid the candy machine.

d. Eat plain protein and vegetables for every meal, skipping most or all starchy vegetables. Buy high-quality plain bittersweet chocolate. After dinner brush your teeth, do all the dishes, and later on sit down with a small piece of the chocolate and savor it slowly.

One Doctor's Natural Treatment for Diabetes

In her family practice at the Community Health Resources Clinic in Philadelphia, Barbara Schneider, M.D., has developed a diet, exercise, and nutritional supplement treatment for diabetes, which is still in the study stage.

Dr. Schneider told me, "The basic diet has 3 servings per day of soy as tofu, soymilk, or beans; 2 servings of broccoli, brussels sprouts, cabbage, kale, turnips, cauliflower, or greens; 2 cloves of garlic; 2 teaspoons of flaxseed; ½ cup of onions; 1 cup of beans or lentils; 1 serving of red grapes; 1 serving of tomato sauce, soup, or fresh tomatoes; 1 serving of yam, sweet potato, mango, carrot, pumpkin, winter squash, papaya, canteloupe, or other orange flesh melon; and 1 serving of blueberries, blackberries, strawberries, cherries, or grapefruit. Servings of a wide variety of fresh vegetables and, to a lesser extent, fruits are added in, according to taste and ethnic background. Whole grains allowed are high beta-glucan (that is, soluble fiber) barley and oats, and a special 70 percent amylose whole grain cornmeal (used in cornbread, grits, and masa harina). Amylose is a starch that is more slowly digested (low on the glycemic index). There are 25 grams of fiber per day in the diet.

"Lean meats used are natural grass-fed beef with 4 percent fat, free-range turkey and chicken breast. Fish or shellfish include tuna, fresh and salt cod, crabmeat, and clams; also salmon is eaten at least weekly. Two to three eggs from free-range hens on special feed are eaten weekly, and skim milk, yogurt, and yogurt cheese are used.

"Fats in the diet are in an n-6/n-3 PUFA ratio of 3.5:1, with 8 percent total saturated fat. The amount of animal fat is low, but it's not absent. Other sources of fat are avocados, olives, walnuts, and their oils, and grapeseed oil. We plan to buy food directly from organic farmers and prepackage some foods for microwave reheating to help some of the elderly."

Dr. Schneider continued with the condiments section: "Red wine; balsamic, white, and cider vinegars; mayonnaise; fish sauce; chicken, beef, and vegetable stocks; and cocoa powder are all used to flavor dishes. Herbs to be consumed daily are parsley, cayenne, cinnamon, mustard, and ginger. Herbs and spices used in ethnic blends include cilantro, oregano, fenugreek, basil, cloves, turmeric, cumin, thyme, sage, bay leaves, burdock, rosemary, dill, nutmeg, tarragon, mints, allspice, black pepper, paprika, and caraway."

The treatment involves important lifestyle changes as well. Dr. Schneider said, "We're using 5 days of exercise: 3 days of 45 minutes walking outdoors or indoors on the Nu-Step machine, and 2 days of 30 minutes Maxercise Super Slow weight training. We have a weekly support group meeting for stress reduction, and also communicate between sessions with e-mail and voice mail. We hope eventually to include the whole family in the program, especially the nutrition and stress reduction parts."

The following supplements are also used:

400 IU mixed tocopherols
Basic B complex
400 mcg folic acid
1,500 mg calcium
400 IU vitamin D
500–1,000 mcg chromium

10

Modern Evolutionary Diet Plan Sample Recipes

Blender Drink Master Recipe

Since this recipe is for a big guy, you may want to halve it, especially if you are consuming it in addition to other food. Made properly, these drinks are complete meal replacements. A professional model Vita-Mix power blender is the best for making blender drinks. Otherwise, use a heavy-duty standing blender with a tight-fitting lid. Hold the lid down with your hand while you run it. Don't use hand-held model blenders. A food processor can be used in a pinch, but does not grind ice well. Place in a blender container the following ingredients:

1. *Cottage Cheese (or substitute):* 1 to 1¼ cup low-fat or nonfat cottage cheese. Other options: plain yogurt, kefir, tofu, or farmer cheese. If you don't want to use these ingredients, double the protein powder.
2. *Protein Powder:* One heaping scoop of protein powder (a measuring scoop is usually enclosed with the protein powder). You can also use ⅓ cup nonfat dry milk or buttermilk powder for all or part of protein powder, but protein powder alone is best.
3. *Fruit:* 1–2 ripe bananas. Keep extra overripe bananas in the refrigerator or freezer. They are great for blender

drinks when all brown and mushy or nearly fermented. Bananas make the smoothest, thickest texture in blender drinks, and are always recommended; however if you don't like them or don't have any around, double the fruits listed below.

In addition to bananas, use 1–2 pieces or 1–1¼ cups any other ripe fruit—what's in season is best. Especially good are mangoes, peaches, pears, nectarines, sweet cherries (pit carefully!), strawberries, ripe papaya, pineapple, and sweeter apple varieties. Like bananas, ripe mangoes make a drink with a superior smooth, thick texture, and so are highly recommended. However, often they need 1–3 weeks of sitting at room temperature to ripen. They must be soft and fragrant to be ripe. Citrus fruits don't work well, and plums, kiwi, and blueberries tend to be too sour, unless they are locally grown or in high season. Sliced whole fresh dates (not the kind that come chopped in a box—they are too hard) or sweet seedless grapes may be used to balance more sour fruits. Also, 1–2 cups of cubed melon of any type can be used, but watch for seeds!

4. *PUFA Oil:* 2 teaspoons flaxseed or Essential Balance oil.
5. *Liquid:* A little water, milk, or juice to assist blending, if needed.
6. *Sweetener:* To taste: stevia, saccharin, aspartame, trutina, maple syrup, molasses, fruit syrup, raw honey, or raw honey with royal jelly. For diabetics, the noncaloric sweeteners stevia, saccharin, or trutina are recommended. You should not need more than two packages of commercial artificial sweetener, ¼ teaspoon of stevia, or 1 teaspoon of trutina. Caloric sweeteners may take up to ¼ cup to satisfy your sweet tooth or balance the sourness of yogurt or fruit. However, caloric sweeteners used judiciously are fine for those who do not need to be concerned about calories, or for children.
7. *Flaxseed Meal:* 2–3 teaspoons (Don't halve this.).
8. *Other Additions:* Good additions are alcohol-free glycerin-

based extracts such as vanilla, almond, maple, or orange, available from health food stores or candy-making suppliers. A small amount of regular ethanol-based extracts can be added, but they tend to be very harsh when overused. Such extracts are designed for cooking and baking, not cold use. Cinnamon, allspice, nutmeg, ginger, or cardamom can be added. You can also use chocolate protein powder and add a heaping tablespoon of cocoa powder for a chocolate blend. Bananas, pears, apples, and sweet cherries go well with chocolate versions, but melons, kiwi, and pineapple are not recommended.

9. *To Make a Creamier Drink: Do before blending!* To add medium chain triglycerides and make the drink really thick and creamy like soft ice cream or a milk shake, add 2–3 teaspoons of coconut oil and blend very well to emulsify coconut oil. Do not add coconut oil after the ice, or it will freeze into a single lump! Alternatively, you may also use 2–4 teaspoons of any nut butter for a nice taste. Creamy commercial peanut butter also makes a nice thick blender drink that appeals to children. You can reduce the PUFA oil by 50 percent if you use nut butter.

Blend all ingredients well. Add a tray or more of ice, and liquid as needed, and blend again until smooth. If you make too much, pour out some "concentrate" into a glass before adding ice, and then blend the rest with ice in two batches. Keep practicing and you will get a number of versions, none necessarily better than the others, just different. The ingredients listed above can be varied to suit your palate, as long as you keep the basic principle of balancing protein, fat, and carbohydrate nutrition.

Other Tips for Thickening: Emulsified coconut oil, flax meal, bananas, mangoes, and of course, ice help thicken blender drinks. Another way to thicken, as well as add soluble fiber, without adding too much ice or fat, is guar gum. Add 1–2 teaspoons of guar gum powder to your mix and blend well prior to adding ice. Be careful, especially when you do add ice, because when it starts to thicken, it can seize up the blender, even the powerful Vita-Mixer. If you use guar gum, start with 1 teaspoon and work up. Guar gum gives superior results if you put the ingredients in the blender, add some water, and let it sit at room temperature for 5–15 minutes. It's a good idea to add the protein powder, extract, guar gum, and some water to the blender and let it sit while you are preparing the fruit.

These drinks are designed for dieters, and so there is not a great deal of fat called for. However, healthful diets are not fat-free. When you start out, don't be exceedingly frugal with fat—make your shakes rich enough so that you do not need to eat ice cream or drink milk shakes. Use lactose-free milk if necessary, and substitute low-fat cream cheese, tofu, kefir, or yogurt for cottage cheese, if it bothers you. The cold-processed whey protein powder I recommend is lactose-free, and tends also to be nonallergenic. This is because the protein in the whey protein powder is mostly in small units called peptides, instead of larger protein units. Peptides tend not to provoke allergic reactions as compared to the larger proteins.

Note: If you use citrus fruits in blender drinks, be sure to remove *all* the white membrane. When this membrane is finely ground, it becomes very bitter. Even a little bit has this effect, and a ground citrus seed can be very bitter also. To prepare oranges and grapefruit, slice rinds down to the bare fruit and section to remove seeds, before putting fruit into blender. Lemons and limes are almost always bitter in blender drinks—use only the juice or an extract if you like this flavor.

Chocolate-Nut Blender Drink

• • •

1–2 ripe bananas

1–2 ripe pears or sweet apples, cored and seeded

1 heaping scoop protein powder, chocolate flavor

1 tbsp flaxseed meal or 2 tbsp pistachio or hazelnut flour

1–2 tbsp peanut butter or other nut butter

½ package sugar-free hot cocoa mix

1 tbsp unsweetened cocoa powder

2 packages saccharin, ⅛ to ¼ tsp stevia powder, or 1 tsp trutina

1 cup fat-free or low-fat cottage cheese (or another scoop protein powder)

2–3 tsp alcohol-free vanilla extract if desired. A small amount of regular vanilla or other extract can be used, but too much will be bitter.

½ cup water

ice, to taste

Blend all ingredients together, adding more water, if needed. Stop blender and add 1 tray ice. Blend in ice. If you want to add more ice or water, pour out some concentrate and then add more ice and continue blending.

Eggnog Blender Drink

• • •

1 ripe banana

1–2 ripe medium mangoes, peeled, or one mango and one apple, peach, pear, nectarine, etc. However, there is no substitute for a good ripe mango in this recipe.

1–2 tsp Essential Balance Jr.™ oil

2–3 tsp coconut oil

1 heaping scoop whey protein powder, vanilla flavor

1–2 tsp flaxseed meal

2 packages saccharin, ⅛ to ¼ tsp stevia powder, or 1 tsp trutina

1 cup fat-free or low-fat cottage cheese, or another scoop protein powder

¼ to ½ tsp alcohol-free butterscotch flavor. This flavor is strong, so do not exceed ½ tsp, but this little bit really makes a professional flavor difference.

¼ tsp (or to taste) ground nutmeg or mace. Start with a little—you can always sprinkle more in, but too much in the blender will be bitter or metallic tasting.

½ cup water or skim milk. Or use whole milk and you will never need to buy ice cream again!

ice, to taste

Blend with same technique as in the master recipe. Make sure that the coconut oil is emulsified before you add ice or it will congeal. Although the mango peels are bitter, they are filled with beneficial phytochemicals, and so I eat the peels while preparing the drink just for the nutrition. Note also that mangoes must be really soft to be ripe. They do ripen off the tree, but can take weeks. Buy the ripest ones you can, and don't refrigerate. I buy a lot of reduced-for-quick-sale fruit because it is very ripe and soft, and hence really sweet and fine to grind up. You don't have to buy fruit for appearance when you are going to grind it up. In season, I also go directly to orchards for peaches, pears, apples, melons, and other fresh fruits in bulk.

Pumpkin Pie Blender Drink

• • •

½ package fat-free cream cheese (I recommend Philadelphia brand. If you have trouble with dairy products, use 1 block of firm tofu instead.)

1 cup canned pumpkin puree

1–2 ripe bananas

1–2 tbsp molasses or dark honey

1 tsp pumpkin pie spice (I mix my own spices here: ginger, cinnamon, cloves, nutmeg—but use whatever you like.)

1 heaping scoop whey protein powder, natural or vanilla flavor

2 tsp flaxseed or Essential Balance oil

2–3 tsp coconut oil or 1 tbsp pumpkin seed butter

1 tbsp flaxseed meal or 2 tbsp hazelnut or almond flour

2 tsp alcohol-free vanilla or maple extract

1 cup water or skim milk (For a treat, try unsweetened evaporated skim milk, or whole milk instead.)

2 packages saccharin, ⅛–¼ tsp stevia powder, 1 tsp trutina

ice, to taste

Blend well. This will be very thick, because of the pumpkin and cream cheese, so make sure to add liquid as needed.

Salmon Spread

• • •

Feed your guests right! This version of this classic, easy, entertaining recipe is filled with balanced n-3 and n-6 PUFA, and good taste too.

1 8-oz package fat-free or reduced-fat cream cheese, softened (I recommend Philadelphia brand.)
3 oz smoked salmon
2 tbsp flaxseed or Essential Balance oil (Try the garlic-chili flavor for a change.)
2 tsp grated horseradish
1–2 tsp fresh lemon juice; or white wine, rice, or cider vinegar

1–2 tsp honey, or 2–3 tsp honey mustard
1½ tbsp chopped fresh dill weed or 1½ tsp dried
⅛ tsp Tabasco
fresh ground black pepper and salt, if needed, to taste
1–2 tbsp milk for adjusting consistency

Place all ingredients, except milk, in work bowl of food processor. Process briefly to blend; scrape down work bowl. Process with long pulses until salmon is coarsely pureed, scraping work bowl as needed. Transfer mixture into small bowl. If serving immediately, adjust consistency if desired by mixing in milk a little at a time. Taste and adjust seasoning also. To serve later, do not add milk, just cover tightly and refrigerate. Let warm slightly before serving and then adjust consistency and seasoning.

Alternatively, salmon may be minced finely with a heavy sharp knife, and all ingredients may be beaten together in a medium bowl with a heavy spoon or spatula. Serve spread on raw vegetables such as cucumbers, carrots, celery, jicama, mushrooms, or thin round oriental rice crackers.

Mexican Coleslaw

• • •

I must have 200 versions of coleslaw that would be great here. This recipe is just a guideline to get you thinking about how you can make this very nutritious staple salad into a version that will reflect whatever type of cuisine you are serving.

2 red bell peppers
1 medium head cabbage
2 carrots
3–5 green onions
handful fresh cilantro
¼–½ cup reduced-fat mayon-
naise
¼–½ cup fat-free sour cream
(I recommend the
Breakstone brand.)
1–2 tbsp garlic-chili-flavored
flaxseed oil

1–3 tbsp red wine, sherry, or
cider vinegar
1–2 tbsp raw honey or
molasses
½–1 tsp ground cumin
¼–½ tsp red chili powder
½ tsp salt
fresh ground black pepper, to
taste
¼–½ tsp sweet paprika, if
desired

Roast red bell peppers by placing on a BBQ grill or under the broiler at medium heat. Roast until skins are blackened, turning from time to time. Allow to cool, then peel and seed. Don't worry if some peel still adheres. Finely chop green onions and red pepper with sharp blade of food processor or knife. Grate cabbage and carrots with food processor shredding disk or grater. Chop cilantro coarsely by hand. Place all vegetables in a large bowl. In a small bowl, whisk together mayonnaise, sour cream, garlic-chili flaxseed oil, honey, vinegar, and spices. Taste and adjust seasonings. Pour dressing over vegetables and blend well. If you are watching your fat intake, you can use the new nearly fat-free mayonnaise, or just be frugal with the amount of dressing you use—but don't neglect your PUFA.

If you love hot spicy food, roast a few fresh hot peppers in the same manner, and chop them up along with the bell peppers. For a terrific taste that no one will identify at first, cut 1 large or 2 small unpeeled onions in half. Roast on the BBQ grill for 15–30 minutes, or until outer skin is blackened and onion flesh is golden and soft in the center. Allow to cool completely. Then chop up with the sharp blade, along with the peppers and green onions. It's a good idea to roast extra onions and peppers to serve hot for one meal, and refrigerate the leftovers to chop up in coleslaw anytime over the next 5 days or so.

Roast Potatoes

• • •

Your whole family, including children, can easily stop eating french fries if you offer this alternative.

3–4 large white or russet potatoes
1–3 tsp cold-pressed peanut, sesame, Brazil nut, or hazelnut oil
½ tsp sea salt (Sea salt really makes a difference here.)

1 tbsp cider or malt vinegar (optional)
garlic powder, paprika, curry powder, rosemary, or hot pepper powder, to taste (optional)

Preheat oven to 400 degrees. Wash and dry potatoes, but do not peel. Slice lengthwise like steak fries or crosswise into ¼–½ inch thick slices. Toss in a bowl with 1–3 tsp oil and sprinkle lightly with sea salt, and spices or vinegar if using, and stir gently to coat evenly. Spread a single layer on a baking sheet. Bake 10 minutes, then turn with a spatula. Don't worry if they stick and break up a bit, just scrape them up. Bake 10–15 minutes longer or until browned, and crisp if you like. Serve immediately. You can't make enough of these—they disappear! Any of the above optional seasonings can be added when you toss the potatoes for a change of pace. Any other seasonings you like, including salt-free blends, also work very well.

Brunswick Stew

• • •

A classic Southern U.S. recipe that originally called for fresh rabbit or squirrel. Many recipes use skin-on chicken and add bacon or salt pork, so we have leaned things out a bit here, but the flavor is still excellent. You can sprinkle on a light topping of crisp-cooked crumbled bacon or turkey bacon as it's served, if you like the smoky flavor and a bit of richness.

2–2 ½ lbs skinless chicken breasts, thighs, or mix; boned or bone in
1 cup white wine
1 cup water
1 tsp salt
1 tsp black pepper
1 tsp or to taste Tabasco
2 medium onions, sliced
1 tsp dried or 2 tsp minced fresh rosemary or thyme

1½ tsp dried or 4 tsp minced fresh basil
2 medium potatoes, peeled and cubed
1 16-oz or slightly larger can crushed tomatoes with juice
1 cup whole kernel yellow corn
1 cup lima beans
1–1½ cups sliced raw okra

Place chicken, wine, water, salt, pepper, onions, Tabasco, and rosemary or thyme in a large pot or Dutch oven. Simmer 30–40 minutes or until chicken is fully cooked. Remove chicken from broth and allow to cool briefly. Bone, if necessary, and shred meat. While chicken is cooling, add cubed potatoes and simmer 7 minutes. Add tomatoes, corn, lima beans, basil, okra, and put shredded chicken back in the pot. Simmer another 20–30 minutes and check seasonings. Add additional Tabasco, salt, or pepper if desired, and serve. This stew is great reheated over the next few days, but does not freeze as well as other stews do.

Turkey Minestrone or
Italian Clam Chowder

• • •

If you like to make homemade soup, here's a basic recipe that adapts soup to the Modern Evolutionary Diet way of thinking, with lots of lean meat and vegetables instead of rice and noodles to fill you up. If you need to have beans in your minestrone, add 1 can drained cooked white or navy beans 10–15 minutes before serving.

2 tbsp extra virgin olive oil
3 medium onions, sliced
3 medium carrots, sliced thinly into disks
3 stalks celery, sliced thinly
2 medium zucchini, sliced or cubed
½ lb Italian pole beans or green beans, cut in 2-in lengths
2–3 cups thinly sliced green cabbage
4 large cloves chopped garlic
6 tbsp tomato paste
3 cups defatted chicken or veal stock

3 cups water, or 2 cups water and 1 cup tomato, carrot, or V-8 vegetable cocktail juice
1 tsp salt (Add more only after tasting finished soup.)
1 tsp black pepper
¾–1 tsp each, dried basil, oregano, and rosemary or savory
¼ cup chopped fresh Italian (flat leaf) parsley
1½ cup diced or shredded cooked turkey
1 cup diced cooked turkey ham or lean ham

Sweat vegetables by placing olive oil, garlic, and all vegetables, except cabbage, in a large soup pot or kettle and placing a sheet of waxed paper over the pot. Cook gently on medium-low heat for 10–15 minutes, stirring occasionally. Do not allow to brown. Next, dissolve tomato paste in 1 cup stock or water, and add to pot along with remainder of stock, water, and juice. Add herbs and spices and simmer 10 minutes. Add cabbage and meat and simmer another 10–30 minutes. Add cooked beans during this time, if using them. Adjust seasonings—since ham may be salty, it is recommended to be frugal with salt prior to finishing soup. A few hot red pepper flakes are a great addition to this soup, as is fresh chopped basil.

To make the clam chowder option, use 1½ lb chopped raw clams with their juice instead of meat, and 2 medium or large diced potatoes instead of the zucchini and green beans. Cut dried herbs, tomato paste, and salt by one-half, and add 1 bay leaf to soup. Use 2 cups water and 2 cups Clamato juice (or 3 water and 1 Clamato); add more water or defatted chicken broth, if necessary, to achieve desired consistency. In this recipe, first make up the whole soup, then add clams to simmering soup just before serving. Simmer only until clams are tender, 6 minutes or less. The same weight of cleaned sliced squid, cubed raw fish, or small peeled raw shrimp can be added instead of or mixed in with clams. Again, cook seafood only until tender—do not overcook or leave soup cooking for second helpings while eating. White or navy beans are not recommended; add lima beans, corn, or an extra potato, if you wish.

Teriyaki Tuna Steaks

• • •

Also great with other firm ocean fish such as mahi-mahi, swordfish, wahoo, or shark.

¹/₃ cup soy sauce
2 tbsp fresh lemon juice, or 1 tbsp lemon juice and 1 tbsp rice vinegar
2 tsp honey or brown sugar
2 tbsp sake, rice wine, or dry sherry
2 tsp minced fresh ginger root
2 medium cloves garlic, pressed or minced (optional)
3–4 tbsp chopped green onion
black pepper, to taste (Add hot pepper powder also, if desired.)
2 lbs fresh tuna steaks

Dissolve honey or sugar in lemon juice (and vinegar, if using) and wine or sherry. Combine rest of marinade ingredients. Taste and adjust flavors: the marinade should taste neither sweet nor sour, just balanced between the two. Rinse fish fillets briefly in cold water, pat dry with paper towels, then place fish in a flat glass or ceramic pan. Pour marinade ingredients over fish, turning fish several times to coat. Marinate up to 45 minutes at room temperature, or 2 hours in the refrigerator, basting and turning from time to time. Grill fish over medium heat about 5–8 minutes per side, or until center of fish is just opaque. Fish does not need to flake easily to be done; it continues to cook off the grill. If using a broiler, set broiler pan on second (not highest) oven rack setting and broil 5–8 minutes per side. Brush green onions off before cooking, as they tend to burn. Serve immediately. Any leftover fish can be refrigerated, and then flaked or sliced for a delicious tuna salad in the next day or two.

If you wish to use this flavor on a more delicate fish, place each fish fillet on a piece of heavy-duty aluminum foil and pour a few tablespoons of marinade over fish. Wrap tightly on both sides, so that you can turn package. Grill foil package over medium heat 6 to 10 minutes per side, or bake at 400 degrees F for 10–15 minutes, depending on thickness of fillets.

Note: It is better to undercook fish than to overcook it. If for example, you pull a tuna steak off the grill and the center is not done but the edges are, 1–3 minutes on high in the microwave will finish the fish beautifully, without drying the edges or burning the marinade, and you will still have the delicious grilled flavor. This tip works well for lean boneless pork and chicken also.

Curry Marinade for Grilled Chicken, Pork, or Firm Fish Steaks

• • •

1 tbsp cold-pressed peanut or sesame oil

1–2 tbsp curry powder, to taste

⅓ – ½ cup plain yogurt, kefir, or low-fat sour cream

¼– ½ tsp black pepper

1 tbsp fresh lemon or lime juice

½ tsp salt

2 cloves garlic, pressed

¼ tsp cayenne or other hot pepper powder

1½ tsp sugar

1–2 tbsp minced fresh ginger root (optional)

1½–2½ lbs skinless chicken, center cut loin or tenderloin boneless pork cutlets, or firm fish steaks

Mix together marinade ingredients in a small bowl and pour over chicken, meat, or fish in a wide glass, ceramic bowl, or flat pan. Turn to coat evenly. Chicken is best if marinated 8 hours or overnight in the refrigerator, stirring from time to time. Grill directly from refrigerator—do not allow marinade to warm up, or it does not stick to the meat as well. Grill chicken over medium or medium-high heat about 10–15 minutes bone down, then 6–10 minutes bone up. Breasts may take longer, but grill for the bulk of the time bone down. Pork can be marinated any length of time over 2 hours. Grill 6–10 minutes per side, or until pork has just a touch of pink in the center. Do not overcook pork or it will be very dry. Marinate fish 2–3 hours only in refrigerator, and then grill or broil as per recipe for the Tuna Teriyaki above.

PART
THREE

Natural Cures
and Prevention

11

Food Allergies and Diabetes

Chronic allergies are one of the major reasons why people turn to natural or alternative medicine for help. When used day after day, antihistamine and decongestant medications lose their effectiveness, and standard treatments such as allergy shots often provide little relief for the amount of time and money spent. People with allergies and asthma are often aware that they must avoid certain foods. They may also have learned to clean up their home and work environments — avoiding perfumes, solvents, mold, dust, pet dander, harsh cleaning products, and so on. Perhaps without even knowing it, they have taken their first steps toward realizing that their allergies are not going to get better simply by using medications that treat the symptoms. A natural approach with a lot to offer emphasizes that you recognize allergens and avoid them, as well as improve your immune system and your overall health. This topic deserves its own book. Here we will discuss only the most important areas of overlap between blood sugar control and food allergies.

As with diabetes, the incidences of chronic allergies, especially asthma, have been increasing steadily in the past 30–50 years, despite continual advances in medical care. Asthma and allergies are strongly linked: most people with asthma have allergies, and allergic reactions are the leading cause of asthma attacks. Asthma is no longer considered a respiratory disease, but rather a chronic inflammatory condition. In this respect, asthma has more in common with arthritis than it does tuberculosis or emphysema. Not many people are aware that, like diabetes and heart disease, asthma is a relatively new disease. It was virtually unknown 100 years ago, is rare in many developing countries, and is more common in urban than rural areas. Childhood eczema and seasonal pollen allergy (hay fever) have also increased in incidence in the past 30 years. Reports of these conditions were much less common at the turn of the century than they are now.

When we see a relatively new disease, we must consider that the very profound changes that have occurred in our diets, lifestyles, and environment in the past 10,000 years since the agricultural revolution, and especially in the past 100–150 years since the industrial revolution, have major roles in the cause of the disease. Although genetic factors may cause you to be more susceptible to a disease or allergy, this susceptibility is activated by the diet or environment. In other words, your body may load the gun, but your environment or your dinner pulls the trigger!

There are two types of food allergies: immediate onset and delayed onset.

Immediate-Onset Food Allergies

Immediate-onset reactions to foods develop minutes or hours after ingesting *any* amount of the allergenic food. Luckily, they are fairly rare, occurring in about 5 percent of the population in Western countries. The characteristic, predictable reactions involving the skin, airway, and gastrointestinal tract are called anaphylaxis. They may include vomiting; diarrhea; mouth; throat, eye, or other tissue swelling; sneezing; wheezing; shortness of breath; bronchospasm; asthma attacks; hives; skin rashes; or fainting. Severe immediate-onset food allergies can cause anaphylactic shock, with respiratory and circulatory failure, convulsions, or cardiac arrest. This type of reaction is similar to the severe allergic reactions caused by insect or poisonous jellyfish stings, and often requires emergency medical treatment or hospitalization. Anaphylactic shock is occasionally deadly. Peanuts are notorious triggers of immediate-onset food allergies, especially in children (usually because adults already know better, since peanut allergies are rarely outgrown). These allergies may be so severe that simply opening a jar of peanut butter and smelling it causes anaphylaxis. Tree nuts, eggs, berries, and shellfish are also frequent causes of severe immediate-onset food allergies.

A child I know with a severe peanut allergy was working on an arts and crafts project in his school classroom that involved making bird feeders. Peanut butter was spread on pieces of wood and birdseeds were pressed into the peanut butter. Although the boy had already twice received emergency medical care at his school after eating peanuts, evidently nobody kept this in mind. He knew better than to lick his fingers, but during the course of constructing his bird feeder, he rubbed his eyes. This caused wheezing, shortness of breath, and eye swelling so severe that he could not see at all, and once again emergency medical treatment was required. Needless to say, his parents were incensed at the school personnel. In some cases, parents have asked entire school classes, airline flights, or church suppers to ban peanut products because of their child's peanut allergy. Currently peanuts are not allowed in my son's preschool class snack time.

Delayed-Onset Food Allergies

These allergies develop a few hours or even 24–48 hours after eating a food, and vary with the amount and preparation of the food eaten. The large variety of responses aren't always predictable or easily linked to the offending food. These responses (as distinct from direct reactions) include stomach cramps, gas and bloating, diarrhea or alternating constipation and diarrhea, migraines or other recurrent headaches, asthma, skin rashes, rheumatoid arthritis, learning disabilities, chronic fatigue, nasal and sinus congestion, recurrent ear infections, pale skin with dark circles under the eyes, abnormally bad premenstrual syndrome, constant runny nose, strong cravings for the same food daily, fluid retention, and obesity. Delayed-onset food allergies are rarely life-threatening. Instead, they tend to turn us into the "walking wounded."

Delayed-onset food allergies are not rare—they are probably very common. We don't know exactly what percentage of the population has them since so few people have had adequate testing for these allergies, and because the allergy is dependent on how much of a food is consumed. However, some doctors believe that more than 50 percent of the population have at least one delayed-onset food allergy. We also know that these allergies are caused by our overexposure to commercial agricultural products. For delayed-onset food allergies, the Top Ten list of allergenic foods reads like the Top Ten list of agricultural commodities, including milk, eggs, soy, and wheat.

Mary is a child I know who had recurrent middle ear infections. After many less-than-successful antibiotic courses, she had ear tubes installed. Unfortunately, her ear problems were not due to recurrent infections *per se,* but rather to an allergy to milk and milk products. The allergies directly caused congestion and the excess fluid aided bacterial proliferation, causing infections to develop. After tubes were installed, her ears drained better, but Mary remained unhealthy, got sick often, and had pollen, dust, and dander allergies. Her immune system was overwhelmed by her constant ingestion of dairy products, and until this burden was alleviated, she did not get well.

In the following lists, the foods on lines marked with an asterisk can cause both immediate and delayed-onset food allergies.

Top Ten Causes of Delayed-Onset Food Allergies

Milk	Cheese, and other dairy products
Wheat, rye*	Baker's and brewer's yeast
Peanuts*	Soybeans*
Eggs*	Corn
Citrus fruits*	Chocolate*

Other Foods That Are Often Allergenic

Fresh tomatoes and tomato sauce products*
Beans and peas (various legumes)*
Fish and shellfish*
Pork and beef
Nuts and cold-pressed nut oils*
Berries, especially strawberries*
Various fruits, especially kiwi, plum, peach, apple, banana, mango, and grape
Various spices, especially black pepper, cayenne, paprika, caraway, ginger, mustard, and poppy seed*
Mushrooms, especially shiitake
Buckwheat, oats, barley
Potatoes
Coffee and malt beverages
Cottonseed meal and oil*
Beer and wine
Condiments: pickles, olives, catsup, mustard, salad dressing, soy sauce, miso, etc.
Artificial colors and preservatives; monosodium glutamate*

Diagnosis of Food Allergies

Immediate-onset food allergies are not so difficult to diagnose. Since the *reaction* to a food is direct, people usually figure out what they are allergic to and learn to stay away from it. Food challenges under medical supervision and skin prick or patch tests can also be used to identify immediate-onset food allergies. Physiologically, immediate-onset food allergies are caused by immunoglobulin E (IgE) antibodies, although some subclasses of IgG may be involved as well. Skin prick tests can identify IgE reactions. To confirm the diagnosis, however, you can eliminate the food from the diet and then reintroduce it in a food challenge. Certainly, severe IgE food allergies do not need any testing to confirm. In fact, tests may induce anaphylaxis, so that testing is not safe unless conducted in a clinic where emergency medical care is available. Cross-reactions can also occur — for example, people allergic to peanuts may also have reactions to a variety of legumes used as foods or herbal supplements. Caution is advised.

In contrast, delayed-onset food allergies may be very difficult to diagnose. Whereas immediate-onset food allergies are usually restricted to one to three foods, delayed-onset allergies may involve three to ten or even twenty foods at once. Physiologically, delayed-onset food allergies are mediated by IgG antibodies, and subclasses IgG_1, IgG_2, IgG_3, and IgG_4 may all be involved. In addition, some of the foods a person is allergic to may produce virtually no symptoms, whereas other foods will produce obvious symptoms. Be that as it may, it is the total load of food allergies that can cause the eventual breakdown of a person's health. Cross-reactions are also common here as well. For example, if you find that kidney beans don't agree with you, eating blackeyed peas and pinto beans instead is no solution, and may eventually cause the same type of response. In these cases, it is necessary to rotate the *entire family* of legumes in and out of the diet every four days or so, and not pick a different bean to eat each day!

For fast, accurate identification of foods that cause delayed-onset responses, I recommend only ELISA (Enzyme Linked Immunosorbent Assay) blood antibody (or antigen) food allergy testing. This state-of-the-art test clearly identifies problem foods and gives you dietary advice to help you avoid or rotate these foods in your meal planning. Skin tests, electrodermal tests, or other such tests are not acceptable for identifying delayed-onset food allergies. In addition, I strongly prefer food allergy testing for all four IgG subclasses. In the ELISA blood test, the antibodies measured reflect a combination of foods you are allergic to and foods you eat fairly often. Even here, though, it is necessary to have some cross-correlation to minimize the occurrence of false positives. For example, if a test gives significant positve reactions to more than thirty foods, the laboratory should redo the test, and if necessary, ask for a new blood draw. People with real allergies to more than thirty foods probably died in childhood! I recommend and use Immuno Labs for blood food allergy testing (for more information, see the Resources section).

Delayed-Onset Food Allergies and Type II Diabetes

Other researchers as well as I have pointed out that Type II diabetes may be linked to food allergies, as follows:

- The Top Ten agricultural foods are the Top Ten allergenic foods. The consumption of a limited number of agricultural foods day after day can cause problems with delayed-onset food allergies.
- Delayed-onset food allergies can in turn cause deficiencies of important nutrients for Type II diabetes prevention, cause abnormal glucose metabolism (either hypo- or hyperglycemia), and often cause obesity as well.
- Over the long term, the allergic load on the immune system and the chronic production of allergic "alarm" chemicals adversely affect the pancreas, as well as reducing the sensitivity of insulin receptors on the cells.
- Chromium deficiency may also develop. Since chromium is already quite poorly absorbed by the body, we simply cannot tolerate further reductions in our capacity to absorb chromium by allergic irritation to our gastrointestinal tract.
- Food allergies may result in immunological changes that cause genetic or other conditions favoring the development of Type II diabetes.

In 1983, Drs. William Phillpott and Dwight Kalita published a popular book in which they attributed (mainly) Type II diabetes to delayed-onset food allergies. They recorded case histories of extreme glucose metabolism abnormalities in patients induced by feeding them certain foods. However, they did not examine the many links between diabetes and straying from the evolutionary diet, and perhaps relied too much on personal anecdotes and unsupported hypotheses. They also wrote at a time when ELISA testing was not readily available, and when the importance of IgG subclasses was not fully defined. For whatever reason, their important observations were almost completely overlooked, even by the alternative medicine community.

In another controlled research study done in 1997, however, Dr. Russell Jaffe found that 13 people with Type II diabetes showed improvements in fasting glucose, glucose tolerance tests, and glycated hemoglobin, and these improvements increased gradually over 6 months when allergenic foods were removed from their diet. Thirteen diabetic control subjects tested positive for food allergies also, but did not have their allergenic foods removed from their diet. The control subjects followed a standard diabetic diet and failed to show any improvements. This objective testing confirmed that the *link* between food allergies and Type II diabetes is real.

If you have Type II diabetes at an unusually young age, are not overweight, or have lost weight and/or started on a treatment plan for diabetes and *not* experienced any improvement in your condition, *please* read this chapter thoroughly and get the appropriate blood tests for food allergies. In fact, everyone with Type II diabetes can benefit from identifying and removing or limiting allergenic foods from their diet. You have very little to lose and much to gain.

What is the number one food you need to avoid whether you get food allergy testing or not? No, it's not sugar, but wheat! I recommend that anyone with or at risk of developing Type II diabetes strongly restrict or completely remove wheat from their diet. I'd extend this precaution to those with Type I diabetes also. (This doesn't mean that sugar is *not* a problem. Please minimize sugar consumption as well.)

Native Americans, for example, have the highest intrinsic incidence of Type II diabetes of any ethnic group, and were not exposed to wheat, rye, barley, or oats until 100 years ago or less—coincidence or cause and effect? Some Native

Americans have made use of corn and other grains such as quinoa for a few thousand years, but most remained hunter-gatherers until recently. Native Americans had no early traditions of baking wheat and barley bread or brewing such as was the case in ancient Sumeria, Egypt, Greece, and Rome. It is estimated that a high percentage of the Native American population has an allergy to wheat. Compared to rice, the other major grain eaten throughout the world, wheat in the form of breads, cereals, and crackers is consistently rated higher on the glycemic index.

Type I Diabetes and Food Allergies

Type I diabetes is also thought to be related to food allergies, but in a somewhat different manner. Type I diabetes is thought to stem from an autoimmune reaction to the pancreas, where the body mistakenly attacks and destroys its own pancreatic cells. In addition, viral infections (such as whooping cough, mumps, hepatitis, and cocksackie) and prolonged use of antibiotics are thought to cause or contribute to Type I diabetes. Those susceptible to autoimmunity, whether genetically or not, may not be able to handle viral infections as well as other individuals, or may have abnormally adverse reactions to antibiotics or vaccines. It has been observed that the incidence of Type I diabetes increases after major influenza epidemics. One way in which lab animals are made diabetic is by exposing them to viral infections or toxins made by bacteria and fungi.

The incidence of childhood Type I diabetes has increased in Western countries in the past 20–30 years. In the Oxford area of England, for example, the total incidence of Type I diabetes in children under 15 increased 4 percent per year from 1985 to 1995, with a huge increase of 11 percent per year in children under age 5. While nobody knows exactly why this increase has occurred, it is thought that allergic reactions to foods introduced early in life may play a role by causing or contributing to autoimmune destruction of pancreatic cells. Breastfed infants, on the other hand, have a significantly lower risk for developing Type I diabetes, even if they are from families considered genetically susceptible. Cow's milk now has caused some controversy. While many researchers believe that IgG reactions to cow's milk aid in the development of Type I diabetes, others do not. Along with milk, though, many researchers implicate wheat, soybean, peanuts, and other legumes as causative factors for Type I diabetes. So, what's the best way to reduce risk? — avoid the most common allergenic foods.

Those with Type I diabetes should definitely get food allergy testing, and the younger the better. If allergenic foods are removed from the diet and aggressive nutritional support is provided early enough in life, the progression of Type I diabetes may be halted before the pancreatic cells are completely destroyed. If you are already an adult, you may be able to improve your condition significantly by removing allergenic foods from your diet. If Type I diabetes runs in your family or you have already had a diabetic child, breastfeed all infants at least 6 months and wean onto formula, if necessary. Do not introduce cow's, goat's, or other milk, soy, peanuts, other legumes, or wheat until after 12–18 months, and then only very carefully. If there are any signs of allergy to these or any other foods, discontinue feeding those foods and seek professional assistance and food allergy testing as soon as possible.

Wheat Intolerance

James Braly, M.D., is an allergy specialist, author, and medical director of Immuno Labs in Fort Lauderdale, Florida. I asked Dr. Braly about the relationship between Type I diabetes and food allergies.

"A link between early introduction of cow's milk products and Type I diabetes does appear to exist," he said. "The milk proteins alpha- and beta-casein, especially alpha-casein, seem to be the most diabetogenic. And other foods are a problem. Soy and wheat are diabetogenic, for example, and exposure to rubella and other viruses is implicated as well.

"Wheat is likely to be a huge problem. When we diagnose and treat people with celiac disease (an extreme inability to tolerate wheat), we're only seeing the tip of the iceberg. Classically, the incidence of celiac disease is 1 in 1,700 people; however, better testing techniques have lowered this to 1 in 200. I would consider it's more like 1 in 85! Currently the incidence of celiac disease is increasing in the Western world, and the way the disease is expressed is changing. The typical symptoms of gastrointestinal irritation are now atypical. Individuals with celiac disease have an increased incidence of thyroid disease (including hyper- and hypothyroid, Grave's disease, and Hashimoto's thyroiditis), Addison's disease, pernicious anemia, and inflammatory bowel disease. Those with Type I diabetes have a tenfold greater incidence of celiac disease—it runs as high as 8 percent of Type I diabetes patients."

Dr. Braly continued, "Authorities are now recommending that anyone with Type I diabetes get tested for celiac disease. If the test is negative, it should still be repeated periodically to make sure that nothing has changed. A set of three out of four possible tests is nearly 100 percent diagnostic; Immuno Labs and other laboratories do these tests for a reasonable cost. Family members of individuals with known celiac disease should also be tested for wheat allergy. And for those that have it, we don't recommend a rotation diet here—wheat needs to be completely removed from the diet. A major reason for this is that the risk for all digestive lymphomas (malignant tumors)—all the way from the mouth to the anus—is 100 times greater in those with celiac disease. However, if wheat is removed from the diet, this risk goes down to zero! Wheat should *not* be removed from the diet prior to the test, though, as this may cause a false negative."

Dr. Braly commented that his mother, now 80, has had Type II diabetes since age 50. She's been keeping it under control with diet, but recently she had been having trouble controlling her blood sugar. Dr. Braly's brothers noticed that she had been eating a lot of wheat products. Upon cutting out the wheat, with no other changes, her blood sugar went from 211 to 141 mg/dl.

Stealth Viruses

Virsuses that adapt to our immune system, thus avoiding destruction by it, do so by stealth. Jeffrey C. Kopelson, M.D., a nutritionally oriented physician in Brewster, New York, thinks it likely that stealth viruses are involved in Type I diabetes, as well as in autism and adult chronic fatigue. According to Kopelson, the stealth virus infection may come first, or perhaps a weakened immune system from other types of previous infections, poor nutrition, or food allergies may allow for later stealth virus infection. Food allergies can also cause the gastrointestinal mucosa to become weakened and more permeable, hence increasing the risk for many types of infections.

I asked Dr. Kopelson whether it was possible that a pre-infection with a stealth virus sets the stage for another factor (such as cow's milk or soybean allergies, childhood vaccinations, or normal viral infections) to "ignite" the chain of events that results in destruction of the pancreatic beta-cells? "Absolutely, this makes sense," he replied. "Dr. John Martin has shown that when cell cultures preinfected with stealth virus are exposed to another virus or a live virus vaccine, there is a tremendous overgrowth of the secondary virus. So a child with a stealth virus may have a very bad reaction to a vaccine, food, or secondary infection—a reaction so bad that the child's immune system is seriously and maybe permanently damaged. This damage may well involve autoimmune destruction of pancreatic cells."

Hypoglycemia Is *Not* the Reverse of Diabetes!

In a small minority of cases, abnormally low blood sugar (hypoglycemia) is due to the side effects of medication or endocrine system abnormalities, such as an overproduction of thyroid or adrenal hormones. But in the vast majority of cases, hypoglycemia is nothing but a *symptom* of delayed-onset food allergies, candida infection, nutrient deficiencies, or simply a diet based far to heavily on carbohydrates. Hypoglycemia is bound to occur when people stray too far from their evolutionary diet, and especially when they base their diet on sugars and refined grains. For example, chromium supplementation has been shown to aid in blood sugar control in people with hypoglycemia as well as diabetes. In these cases, it might be that when chromium is deficient, insulin is overproduced after food is consumed, causing the blood sugar to drop precipitously. This would be similar to the effect when a person with Type I diabetes overdoses on an insulin injection. Since chromium is a cofactor for insulin and apparently improves insulin efficiency, supplementing chromium in hypoglycemics allows for less insulin to do the same job, thus normalizing the system.

Checklist for Anyone with Hypoglycemia

1. See your doctor to rule out any medical conditions.
2. Follow the Modern Evolutionary Diet *closely*.
3. Get ELISA food allergy testing.
4. Follow the basic nutritional supplement plan *closely*.
5. Consider that you may have a candida or, possibly, a parasitic infection.

Polysystemic Chronic Candidiasis (PCC)

If hypoglycemia, multiple allergies, chronic fatigue, chemical sensitivities, yeast or fungal infections, adult-onset asthma, gas, bloating, or cramps after meals, anal itching, heavy mucus drainage, sinusitis, skin rashes, or mystifying chronic health conditions have been plaguing you for a while, you may have PCC. PCC is a yeast infection "gone wild," infecting any or all of the tissues in your body. Candida yeast, of course, is always present in our colon; when it goes wild though it can proliferate throughout the gastrointestinal system, entering the vagina or penis and scrotum, or the bloodstream, affecting many body tissues. Even if an overgrowth is restricted to the colon, toxic metabolic products from the yeast's growth end up in the bloodstream, causing illness. High-carbohydrate diets, use of antibiotics, steroids, and oral contraceptives, alcoholism, nutrient deficiencies, starvation or wasting diseases such as AIDS and cancer, and preexisting food allergies can all cause or contribute to PCC.

We all have symbiotic bacteria in our intestines, which aid our digestion. Candida yeast is also present, and is usually benign. The overuse of antibiotics consistently kills the beneficial bacteria, allowing candida yeast to proliferate to an unnatural degree. This proliferation may be aided by high sugar and starch diets, and lack of certain vitamins, trace elements, food compounds, and PUFA. The yeast growth further irritates the gastrointestinal system, causing poor absorption of nutrients. This malnutrition weakens the immune system, causing even worse allergy and chronic infection problems, such as ear infections and colds.

In addition, the yeast can cause the intestinal wall to weaken, a condition called mucosal hyperpermeability. Lack of PUFA, protein, and the amino acid glutamine contribute to this condition. When the intestinal wall grows too permeable, it allows more and larger molecules of allergenic foods to enter the bloodstream, where they cause even worse allergic reactions. New allergies and chemical sensitivities can thus arise, *directly weakening* the immune system. The result is more congestion, more antibiotics, even more yeast growth and worse allergies in a downward spiral. Yeast proliferation also interferes with neurological functioning and normal appetite. Terrible mood changes, lack of concentration, headaches, urogenital infections, rashes, chemical sensitivity, indigestion, bloating, sinusitis, cravings for sugar and starch, chronic fatigue, *and hypoglycemia* can occur.

The yeast eats sugar and alcohol, and the more it grows, the hungrier it is. However, as the yeast proliferates, allergies and nutrient absorption get progressively worse, and blood sugar levels may drop routinely. People begin to crave sugar and refined starches for their "instant energy" effect, but these foods are feeding the yeast, not you! PCC is a disease caused by straying from our evolutionary diet. In a diet without grains, sugar, beans, fruit juice, alcohol, and dairy products, both carbohydrate intake and delayed-onset food allergies are strongly reduced. Women taking oral contraceptives need to be aware of their increased susceptibility to yeast infections, and take appropriate measures to prevent the initial candida overgrowth.

Getting Rid of Candida

If you suspect PCC, you should see a qualified practitioner for help. However, if you understand that, just like Type II diabetes, hypoglycemia and PCC are overwhelmingly modern diseases brought on by straying from the evolutionary diet, there is no need to follow any complicated diet plans or use unproven supplements or bizarre natural medications (like colloidal silver!). Here's a simple checklist for conquering candida.

1. Follow the Modern Evolutionary Diet and supplement plan perfectly. If you are very ill, avoid dairy products (some cultured dairy products such as kefir might be all right), restrict fruits to grapefruit, and eat only small portions of

starchy vegetables *always* with protein and fat. You will feel awful for the first few days, but just live through it. Take 1,000 mg of vitamin C and a capsule of Siberian, Korean, or American ginseng every 3 hours, and a high potency mutivitamin daily for your "carbohydrate withdrawal." Use valerian, kava-kava, passion flower, or blends containing these herbs at night, if you can't sleep.

2. Get ELISA blood food allergy testing and an accurate blood candida test also.

3. Get a refillable prescription antifungal drug. I prefer fluconazole (Diflucan) in a 150 mg dose per week for 6–8 weeks, or in more serious cases, 50–300 mg per day or every other day for 10–30 days. However, I am not a medical doctor, and so you will need to find an open-minded doctor to help you get the right prescription for your individual case. He or she may also wish to combine antifungal medications for you.

4. My top botanicals for candida eradication are flaxseed meal (2 tablespoons per day, mixed in water), *Pseudowintera colorata*, oregano oil, santolina oil, Pau D'Arco, grapefruit seed extract, coptis, and some other Chinese herbs used in blends. Use botanical supplements as directed by the manufacturer (see the Resources section for more information).

5. Probiotic supplementation.

6. Take 10–20 grams of glutamine powder mixed in water daily. Drop to every 3 days after you are feeling better.

7. If you can, repeat food allergy testing after 6–12 months, or when you're much better. Some of your food allergies may be due to PCC. These will diminish in intensity or leave entirely as you heal.

12

Medicinal Plants for Diabetes

We've talked a lot about how present-day sources and amounts of protein and fat have changed dramatically from our evolutionary diets, but what about plant foods? Our ancestors ate a variety of fresh, wild vegetables, fruits, nuts, and seeds. This is a far cry from today's heavy reliance on a handful of major agricultural crops. The overwhelming majority of plant foods in our diet come from only wheat, white rice, sugar, and corn syrup. These foods, as well as many other cereal grain and legume foods, are concentrated sources of carbohydrates but dilute sources of protein and trace nutrients.

We've discussed how junk food and refined processed foods (especially carbohydrate foods) lose a large percentage of their vitamins and trace elements. This leads to nutrient cannibalization—the situation where the food eaten does not even provide the nutrients necessary to metabolize the calories in the food. Nutrient cannibalization is applicable to phytochemicals, too. Our ancestors' diets were exceedingly rich in phytochemicals compared to our diets today, and we have come to realize that humans literally evolved "bathed" in these phytochemicals. It is quite likely that we are adapted to having these compounds in our diet, and our good health depends in part on their presence. Jim Duke, Ph.D., and I were some of the first scientists to broadly publish and lecture on this concept, and there seems to be more and more converts every day.

Research study after research study has come to the same conclusion: The higher the consumption of fruits and vegetables in the diet, the lower the risk for *any* chronic disease, from diabetes to cancer. Conversely, those who eat few fruits and vegetables are more prone to disease and more likely to die prematurely. A single, particular phytochemical does not necessarily prevent or cure a disease; rather, the absence of a broad range of plant phytochemicals in the diet brings on the disease.

Many biochemically active phytochemicals belong to groups known as flavonoids, saponins, alkaloids, lignans, and tannins. These compounds are usually bitter or astringent. Therefore, horticulturists have bred plants to contain low levels of them or concentrate them in peels that are not eaten. Produce is consistently bred to be larger, sweeter, and milder. The fruits and vegetables our Paleolithic ancestors ate were more akin to chickweed, choke cherries, and kumquats than iceberg lettuce, bing cherries, and navel oranges! Consequently, we have lost a good deal of phytochemical protection from many diseases, diabetes included. The blander and more processed the diet, the greater the loss.

The strong-tasting vegetable kale, for example, had the highest antioxidant capacity of 21 vegetables tested in a research study. This is not surprising, since wild kale is the precursor to all cruciferous vegetables, from kohlrabi to cabbage to cauliflower. Kale bears the most similarity to the cruciferous vegetables that we evolved eating.

Many of these bitter and astringent phytochemicals are with us today in the form of herbal products. The use of medicinal plants for diabetes is not just a search for safer alternatives to pharmaceutical drugs. Herbs can return valuable components to our diet, thereby making it more similar to our evolutionary diet, with a minimum of effort or bad taste.

Over 200 pure phytochemicals are known to be hypoglycemic, but many (and the plants containing them) are dangerous because they are toxic to our metabolisms or liver. Conversely, there are hypoglycemic plants which are very safe and effective precisely because they help return us to our evolutionary diet. And it is these plants that we will focus on in this chapter.

Bitter Melon and Jackass Bitters

I asked Dr. James Duke to tell me about some of the herbs that he has seen used successfully for diabetes. He replied, "Few herbs have attracted as much interest as the food plant known as balsam pear or bitter melon (*Momordica charantia*). Research on its hypoglycemic properties was first published in India in the 1960s, and in a recent trial a fall of 54 percent in blood sugar was achieved. Bitter melon juice, dried fruits, and seeds have proven oral hypoglycemic activity, due to several identified compounds. The researchers recommend 2 ounces of fresh juice or a 100 ml decoction (chop 100 grams of fresh fruit and boil in 200 ml of water down to 100 ml).

"In another study, consumption of 50 ml extract of bitter gourd reduced hyperglycemia by some 20 percent. Bitter melon was shown to delay the development of cataracts and other diabetic complications in rats. Dr. H. F. Dankmeijer of Bilthoven uses bitter melon as an insulin substitute in insulin-dependent diabetics. In Type II diabetes, where insulin resistance is the problem, treatment consists of liver-cleansing agents such as *Milkthistle*, *Chelidonium* (celadine), and *Taraxacum* (dandelion), all of which have been cited as food plants elsewhere. I'd be reluctant to eat much *Chelidonium*. Better yet, just eat it as a side dish, like the Asians and Indians do."

I asked Dr. Duke about herbs that haven't gotten into the mainstream yet. He said, "Central American herbal expert Dr. Rosita Arvigo and I have listed a whole host of ailments treatable with jackass bitters (*Neurolaena lobata*): amoebas, beef worm, candida, other fungi, giardia, headlice, intestinal parasites, ringworm, and screwworm.

As a matter of fact, Rosita sells jackass bitters as the primary ingredient of her Traveler's Tonic for tourists suffering from Montezuma's revenge or malaria. Rosita also stresses the power of jackass bitters for vaginal yeast infections.

"But none of this anticipates what may be the most promising activity of jackass bitters — its antidiabetic activity," Dr. Duke continued. "In my files at the USDA is a copy of a 1989 letter from a Florida physician to the then director of the USDA Beltsville Human Nutrition Research Center, Dr. Walter Mertz: 'Enclosed is a sample of "weed" provided to me by a diabetic patient. This is a rather interesting adult-onset diabetic who had been insulin-requiring until beginning this weed. The patient brought back this weed from Trinidad. I am hoping you will be able to identify the plant and to determine its effective ingredient.' The patient reported that she mixed a small portion of the weed with vermouth and took small sips of this about twice a day. This resulted in normalization of her blood sugar over approximately six months. Knowing of my interest in folk medicine, Dr. Mertz sent me the letter and specimen, which I tentatively identified as jackass bitters, since only leaves had been submitted.

"Research has confirmed the antidiabetic activity of jackass bitters. A 100 percent ethanol extract (a bit stronger than vermouth!) is antihyperglycemic (prevents high blood sugar) in mice orally at doses of 250 mg per kilogram. If I were a 110-kilogram mouse, that would mean I'd have to drink 27.5 grams of nearly 200 proof jackass vermouth (less than a single-ounce shot). A double-shot dose (500 mg/per kg orally in the mouse) certainly lowers blood sugar."

Actions of Phytochemicals Against Diabetes

Hypoglycemic Action. In some cases, phytochemicals can directly stimulate insulin secretion, or improve insulin action and binding. Cinnamon, cloves, and green and black tea have been shown to have an insulin-potentiating or insulin-like action in cell cultures. It was thought at first that these spices might have high chromium concentrations, but measurements showed no correlation between chromium and insulin activity. This means that the spices have an intrinsic hypoglycemic (blood-sugar-lowering) effect. Juniper berries, Siberian ginseng, ganoderma mushroom, cumin, cucumber, and bottle gourd have shown hypoglycemic activity in animal tests. The table at the end of this chapter lists some of the more promising hypoglycemic plants that have not yet been adequately tested in humans.

Improving Muscle Capillary Function. A lean person who exercises has little marbling fat and good circulation of blood to the muscles. Consequently, he or she tends to have more efficient glucose metabolism and a lesser risk for diabetes. A sedentary fat person has much more marbling fat and poorer blood circulation to the muscles, and hence has less efficient glucose metabolism and a greater risk for diabetes.

Anyone, including the sedentary fat person, can improve his or her circulation to some degree by simply taking advantage of herbs that can improve the function of the capillaries (smallest blood vessels) within the skeletal muscles. Examples of such herbal products are horse chestnut, bilberry, ginkgo biloba, gotu kola *(Centella asiatica)*, and various standardized anthocyanin preparations (for example, grape seed and grape skin extract, pycnogenol, and pine bark extract). Bilberry, in particular, has been shown to improve edema (excessive, chronic fluid retention due to poor circulation) and blockage and hardening of capillaries in diabetics. Buckwheat, butcher's broom, or the phytochemical hydroxyethyl rutoside significantly regressed diabetic retinopathy (deterioration of the retina of the eye), lowered total cholesterol and triglycerides, and raised HDL cholesterol.

Antioxidant Action. Botanical antioxidants can play a role in diabetes by helping to maintain the integrity of cell membranes by preventing oxidative damage to PUFA, known broadly as peroxidation. Cloves, cumin, cinnamon, curcumin (turmeric), rosemary, oregano, and many mints are powerful antioxidants, synergistic with each other and with antioxidant vitamins and trace elements. For example, dried ground and fresh spices were found to be highly effective at preventing lipid peroxidation of cooked ground fish. The order of effectiveness for dried spices was: cloves, cinnamon, cumin or black pepper, fennel or fenugreek; for fresh juice, it was turmeric or ginger, garlic, and onion. Fatty acid peroxidation and damage by reactive oxygen species are also major problems in terms of diabetic complications, and are discussed further in Chapter 13.

Herbs for Treatment of Diabetes

Some antidiabetic herbs have been proven effective in controlled human studies. In all cases, these herbal products cannot be expected to reverse diabetes alone, but are to be used as adjuncts to diet, exercise, and nutritional supplementation. You need to experiment on yourself with different herbs to see which work for you. It also helps to stick with brand-name herbs from leading manufacturers to make sure you are getting effective products. Some of the companies that I use and recommend are listed in the Resources section.

Bitter Melon (Momordica charantia)

Unripe bitter melon is used traditionally in India, Africa, and Asia as a diabetic remedy and bitter tonic food. It is available in most Asian groceries. Bitter melon contains a mix of hypoglycemic compounds called charatin, with an insulin-like protein. The effects of bitter melon are gradual and cumulative.

A juice or decoction has been shown to be effective, but crude preparations of dried herb have not. A decoction is made by pouring boiling water over chopped fresh fruit, steeping, and straining.

Eat cooked sliced bitter melon with one or two meals per day, or drink the decocted juice as described above. You may need to start with only a few slices or 50 ml of juice and work up to 200 ml after 3 weeks. Use 200 ml for 4 weeks or so, and monitor your progress. Then adjust your dosage down to an effective maintenance dosage. This gradual procedure is the approach to take for both types of diabetes.

Alternatively, a standardized encapsulated bitter melon extract is now available. Start with two capsules per day and increase slowly to four to six capsules per day (see the Resources section).

Gurmar (Gymnena sylvestre)

The leaves of this climbing vine comprise an ancient Ayurvedic treatment for diabetes. Gurmar appears to stimulate insulin secretion, and lowers cholesterol and triglycerides without side effects. It has been shown to rejuvenate dysfunctional pancreatic cells in diabetic rats. In an open study in India, gurmar was tested on 22 patients who were not insulin dependent but taking oral antidiabetic medications. The patients were given 400 mg of a standardized gurmar extract per day for 18 to 20 months. They were all able to reduce their medication dosages, and 5 were able to discontinue their medications. The extract was judged superior to the medications for long-term blood sugar stabilization, lowering of triglycerides, and the overall well-being of the patients. In a sister controlled study, 400 mg of the extract was given to 27 insulin-dependent diabetics. Insulin requirements dropped by nearly 50 percent, and fasting blood sugar dropped also. Triglycerides dropped to near normal levels, and the subjects reported that their mood and physical performance improved.

Since gurmar acts primarily to increase insulin secretion, it may not be appropriate for individuals with chronically high levels of circulating insulin. This would include most people with Type II diabetes, but nobody with Type I diabetes. In fact, gurmar is an herb that is probably targeted more toward those with Type I diabetes than those with Type II diabetes. Gurmar does not seem to lower blood sugar levels in all people and takes time to become effective, but the beneficial effects on triglycerides and cholesterol may make it worth trying no matter what. One capsule of a standardized extract can be taken 1–4 times per day. Those with Type I diabetes or on diabetic medications should start with 1 capsule per day and increase by 1 capsule per week, monitoring blood sugar closely.

Korean ginseng (Panax ginseng)

Traditional Chinese medicine recognized that ginseng helped diabetes centuries ago. On the Western side of the globe, a landmark 1995 Finnish study of diabetics found that only 200 mg of ginseng per day for 8 weeks improved mood and physical activity, and lowered fasting blood glucose and body weight compared to a placebo.

This is only a very small ginseng dosage, and I would not hesitate to recommend 200 mg of ginseng extract or 500 mg capsules, 2–4 per day. Those with Type I diabetes or on diabetic medications should start with 1 capsule and increase by 1 capsule per week, monitoring blood sugar closely; however, dramatic changes in glucose should not be expected. Excessive amounts of Korean ginseng may cause elevated blood pressure, so you should check your blood pressure periodically while increasing your dosage. However, I believe that the benefits from such a safe, time-tested herb far outweigh the risks.

Onions and Garlic (Allium cepa, Allium sativum)

Onions and garlic both contain two chemicals with sulfur-sulfur bonds. Insulin has a similar bond, and the compounds in onions and garlic are thought to bind to enzymes that serve to inactivate insulin, thereby prolonging the life of an insulin molecule. A 1989 study reported that 10 grams per kilogram of body weight of onion or garlic extract lowered fasting blood glucose and improved glucose tolerance by 7–18 percent. This is quite a lot—a kilo of onion or garlic extract per day for a 100-kilo man! Garlic is also an antioxidant and can lower cholesterol significantly.

An extensive review found that somewhat lower doses of garlic are effective; however, most of the studies cited are old, uncontrolled research. Newer studies indicate that the sulfur-containing phytochemical s-allycysteine sulfoxide (alliin) may be important for garlic's effectiveness. Garlic and onion oils contain the majority of this phytochemical.

In one double-blind study, 10 subjects were given 800 mg of garlic per day for 4 weeks. The garlic tablets were standardized for their alliin content. Those receiving the garlic significantly lowered their fasting blood glucose. In another study, spray-dried garlic powder (which does not contain alliin) was given at 700 mg per day for a month, and had no effect.

The bottom line is that onions and garlic are known treatments for diabetes, and are probably helpful, but do not approach the effectiveness of other antidiabetic herbs and foods. Use them as adjuncts to other herbal and nutritional treatments. If it suits you, it's good practice to eat onions, garlic, leeks, shallots, or chives on a daily basis. Raw would be your first choice, then very lightly cooked. Otherwise you might want to take up to 8 standardized garlic capsules per day.

Holy basil (Ocimum sanctum)

In a study at MS University of Baroda in India, 12 male and 5 female Indian diabetic patients were supplemented with 1 gram of dried powdered holy basil leaf per day for 30 days. Supplements were taken once in the morning on an empty stomach, and 5 male and 5 female diabetic patients served as controls, receiving no supplementation. All subjects were taking oral hypoglycemic medications and remained on the same diet throughout the study. Holy basil supplementation lowered fasting blood glucose 20.8 percent, glycated proteins

(for example, hemoglobin) 11.2 percent, total plasma cholesterol 11.3 percent, LDL cholesterol 14.0 percent, and triglycerides 16.4 percent. There was no change in HDL cholesterol.

The researchers noted that 70 percent of the essential oil of
holy basil leaves is eugenol—an effective fat-soluble antioxidant—and which may provide some protection to beta-cells
in the pancreas. Saponins may exert a cholesterol-lowering
effect in concert with other phytochemicals present in the
leaves. As only a few percent of the leaves is essential oil, most
important here are these other yet unknown phytochemicals.
Certainly, more research is called for, as the patients were not
taken off medications, and it may be that basil simply potenti-
ated the drug effects. Nonetheless, holy basil is a safe food
plant, and I don't hesitate to recommend 1–2 grams per day.

Insulin Resistance

Tim Birdsall, N.D., considered an expert in the natural
treatment of Type II diabetes, told me: "My Type II diabetes patients and others who are not yet diagnosable as
diabetics all have insulin resistance (IR) in common. I see
degrees of IR and overt diabetes as different points along
the same line. In most cases, IR stems directly from inactivity and a diet too high in carbohydrates. I recommend
higher protein, lower carbohydrate diets for diabetes and
IR. It's also important to realize that 20–40 percent of all
adults may have IR. They don't yet have diabetic symptoms, but if they don't change their diet and lifestyle, they
soon will. So these principles actually apply to a lot of us!"

Dr. Birdsall says that for Type II diabetes patients, he
tends to use nutritional supplements first, to see how
they work, and then moves on to botanicals if needed.
This stands in contrast to his treatment for Type I diabetes, in which he uses botanicals and supplements con-
currently from the beginning. He prefers to use a fairly
large number of supplements, but I asked him to reduce
them to "must-haves"—that is, supplements that you

can't do without if you have Type II diabetes and aim to reverse it. He recommends taking the following daily:

Vitamin C: 3–6 grams.
Vitamin E: 800 IU.
Chromium: Start with 1,000 mcg per day and adjust the dosage as needed.
Magnesium: 500–1,000 mg per day.
Alpha lipoic acid: around 500 mg per day.

His top recommended botanical supplements are gymnema, bilberry, and gingko. He uses gingko mainly to help treat neuropathy.

Dr. Birsdsall sets ground rules for losing body fat. "Most of my Type II diabetes patients have too much body fat, but this is to a large degree due to their IR," he said. "IR causes you to gain fat, and makes it harder to lose the fat that you already have. Normalizing IR is the biggest single step in losing fat. Fat comes off naturally, or at least the gaining stops, when IR is treated. Exercise is the single most important factor in burning stored fat and it also improves IR. Of course, IR is also improved through diet and supplements. If excess body fat is a problem and people need something to help motivate them, I use a combination of ephedra and white willow for its thermogenic effect. I use it only with caution, and in patients who agree to start an exercise program as well. It can give patients an initial push toward their goal, which helps motivate them. I don't use vanadyl sulfate for everyone, but this type of very overweight patient seems to benefit from it."

Beyond Fiber: Diabetes Treatment and Prevention

High-fiber diets are uniformly recommended for treatment of both Types I and II diabetes. Particularly important is soluble fiber, found mainly in fruits, vegetables, and some seeds. Insoluble fiber is more characteristic of brans and husks of whole grains (wheat bran, bran cereal, brown rice). Soluble fibers include pectins, gums, and mucilages, all of which tend to increase the viscosity of food in the intestine, thus slowing or reducing the absorption of glucose. If you think of how pectin gels a fruit syrup into jelly, which is still soft but definitely not liquid, you can imagine how soluble fiber might act in your intestines.

In this respect, any diet featuring large quantities of raw or lightly cooked vegetables is beneficial for diabetics, especially Type II. Not surprisingly, our evolutionary diet was extremely high in vegetables and soluble fiber; however, people today often shun vegetables rich in soluble fiber, such as okra, turnips, and parsnips. Many herbs and foods with a good deal of pectin or mucilage have also been used successfully for diabetes, along with their soluble fiber content. In fact, epidemiological studies have shown that diets rich in whole grains, fruits, and vegetables result in a decreased incidence of Type II diabetes in a given age group, as opposed to diets rich in white flour, white rice, other refined grains, and sugars. Know this, though: There's more to certain herbs than a simple inhibition of glucose absorption. The following herbs, shown to be effective in human studies and clinical treatment, go well "beyond fiber," providing synergistic benefits beyond the physical effect of simply inhibiting glucose absorption.

Flaxseed (Linum usitatissimum)

Flaxseed meal (food-grade flaxseed with most of the oil pressed out) is one of the richest sources of fiber. In a University of Toronto study, 5 nondiabetic subjects were given a glucose solution, along with plain water or water containing mucilage extracted from flaxseed. The flaxseed mucilage dose improved glucose tolerance by 27 percent compared to the water. Two other groups were given either plain white bread or bread with 25 percent flaxseed meal. The flaxseed bread improved glucose tolerance by 28 percent compared to plain bread. Since the mucilage content of flaxseed meal is only a few percent, there must be more going on than simple inhibition of glucose absorption. Flaxseed is the world's richest source of lignans and also has protein, PUFA, and trace minerals, all of which are evidently beneficial.

Use of flaxseed meal is described in the Diet Plan. Properly used, flaxseed meal is probably the easiest and most effective herbal treatment. Three to nine teaspoons of flaxseed meal can be used per day with no gastrointestinal discomfort. For both Types I and II diabetes, start with 1 teaspoon of flaxseed meal twice per day and increase to 3 teaspoons twice per day. Make sure that you mix the flaxseed meal with water or another liquid, or cook with it—do not consume it dry. (See the Resources section for a recommended supplier.)

Fenugreek (Trigonella foenum-graecum)

Fenugreek is another Ayurvedic tradition that has proved effective. Whole fenugreek seeds are about 50 percent fiber, with 20 percent of that mucilage. In a double-blind study by the Indian National Institute of Nutrition, 10 Type I diabetes patients were given meals with 100 grams of fenugreek powder (ground defatted, debitterized seeds) per day or regular meals. After 10 days, fasting glucose decreased by 30 percent, and glucose tolerance improved in those that had fenugreek. The amount of sugar excreted in their urine dropped an astonishing 54 percent, yet there was no increase in insulin levels. Since fasting glucose was strongly affected, simple inhibition can't be the only explanation. In addition to mucilage, fenugreek also contains protein, saponins, and the hypoglycemic phytochemicals coumarin, fenugreekine, nicotinic acid, phytic acid, scopoletin, and trigonelline. In other double-blind studies, 15–25 grams of fenugreek powder were similarly effective for Type II diabetes patients. In all studies, fenugreek was very effective at lowering LDL cholesterol and triglycerides.

Fenugreek at only 5 grams daily was also given to 20 patients with Type II diabetes, but no coronary artery disease, for 1 month. Ten patients had severe diabetes, and 10 had mild diabetes. Two groups of 10 mild to severe Type II diabetes patients served as controls. Fenugreek lowered fasting and post-meal blood sugar, but changes were significant only in the mild Type II diabetes group. This indicates that 5 grams may be a preventive dose, while larger daily doses are needed to treat or reverse Type II diabetes.

Fenugreek powder is available in bulk in Indian groceries or from the bulk spice supplier listed in the Resources section. You can also buy whole seeds in bulk and grind them yourself in a spice mill or coffee grinder. Start with ¼ teaspoon stirred in a glass of water 3 times per day, and increase to a heaping teaspoon 3 times per day. Fenugreek at these levels may cause flatulence. If this bothers you, lower your dosage and combine fenugreek with other herbs. You may want to stick to eating weekly curries instead!

Alternatively, a standardized fenugreek fiber extract is available, which is designed to be effective at 5–10-gram doses. (See the Resources section for a recommended supplier.)

Nopal (Prickly Pear Cactus) (Opuntia spp.)

Widely used as a food throughout Latin America, nopal is rich in pectin. In a Mexican hospital study, 8 diabetics were given 500 grams of nopal on an empty stomach. Five tests were performed on each subject, 4 with different cooked or raw cactus preparations and 1 with water. After 180 minutes, fasting glucose was lowered by 22–25 percent by all of the nopal preparations, as compared to 6 percent for water. In a study on rabbits, nopal improved tolerance of injected glucose by 33 percent (180-minute value is also given for comparison) as compared to water. In both these cases, there was no glucose in the intestines, so it's apparent that there's more to nopal, too.

To use nopal, purchase the fresh cactus from a grocery with a Latin American produce section and eat a cup cooked or raw every day. Canned nopal is also widely available. Most Safeways in larger metropolitan areas, for example, have nopal. Dried nopal preparations have not been shown conclusively to be effective, but encapsulated products are now available, and may soon be standardized. Alternatively, delicious prickly pear salsas are available by mail order from Arizona (see the Resources section for a recommended supplier).

Ivy Gourd (Coccinia indica)

In a double-blind study of 32 Pakistani diabetics, 6 tablets of ivy gourd leaves per day for 6 weeks decreased fasting glucose and improved glucose tolerance by 20 percent. Although ivy gourd is rich in pectin, it also helps inhibit the manufacture of glucose by the liver, and stimulates the use of glucose for energy. Ivy gourd is not generally available in the North American marketplace, but it may be in the future, or other plants similar to it will be offered based on newer research.

Other plants known to have the antidiabetic "soluble fiber plus" synergy are aloe vera, Indian cluster bean, and carrots. Undoubtedly there are more.

Ayurvedic Herbs for Diabetes

Vladimir Badmaev, M.D., Ph.D., of the Sabinsa Corporation in Piscataway, N.J., is a pathologist and immunopharmacologist. Sabinsa specializes in standardized extracts of Ayurvedic botanicals.

Dr. Badmaev talked to me about bringing some of the ancient traditions up to speed. "At this point, Ayurveda has more potential treatments for diabetes than any other system of traditional medicine," he said. "Fenugreek lowers blood glucose and lipids, but the doses of ground fenugreek seed needed have a side effect, too— distinctive flatulence! Sabinsa has developed Fenufibers, a defatted fiber-rich fraction of fenugreek seeds that is effective at lower, realistic doses—about 5 to 10 grams per day. Defatted fenugreek fiber concentrate is the form that has shown the best results in research studies also. Fenufibers is useful for both Type I and Type II diabetics.

"We also manufacture standardized *Gymnema, Momordica* (bitter melon), and *Tinospora* (guduchi) products, all of which are primarily for clinical treatment of Type II diabetes. These products should reduce some of the guessing-game nature of applying the ancient herbal medicines, and give any open-minded practitioner an incentive to try Ayurvedic herbs for diabetes and its many complications."

Dr. Badmaev continued, "*Tinospora cordifolia* is another herb that looks promising for the future. It has performed well in animal studies, and was a component of an Ayurvedic formulation tested on 43 Type II diabetes patients. The patients were given a combination of *Tinospora cordifolia, Pterocarpus marsupium, Ficus glomerulata, Momordica chantaria, Ocimum sanctum,* and *Gymnema sylvestre* for 12 weeks. It was found that oral diabetic medications could be omitted in 80 percent of the cases, and insulin administration could be safely reduced in patients who were otherwise stabilized."

Cinnamon

In the laboratory where I work at the U.S. Department of Agriculture, we have investigated over 60 plant extracts in a special cell culture test that determines how much a particular compound stimulates the uptake and utilization of glucose. While these tests are no substitute for human or animal studies, they are important because they identify safe compounds that act directly on cell metabolism. Plenty of plants and individual phytochemicals can lower blood sugar, but many accomplish this by imposing toxic effects on the body. Cinnamon was by far the most active compound in our assay, so we focused on it. From an extract of commercial cinnamon, we identified new phytochemicals called chalcone polymers that increase glucose metabolism in the cells twentyfold or more.

In addition, cinnamon contains anthocyanins of the type thought to improve capillary function, and an extract similar to ours has been shown to inhibit the formation of ulcers and increase blood flow to the stomach in rats. As chalcone polymers strongly inhibit the formation of reactive oxygen species in activated blood platelets, we also know them as antioxidants. A number of antioxidant phytochemicals have already been identified in cinnamon, so that cinnamon may have all three of the beneficial actions mentioned previously.

Since the first published results that identify cinnamon as a potential therapy for diabetes, we have heard from hundreds of people who found that it works. Since cinnamon is very safe, there is little harm in trying it yourself. To use cinnamon to help lower blood sugar and broadly improve Types I and II diabetes, put 3 rounded tablespoons of ground cinnamon and ½–1 teaspoons of baking soda (use a lesser amount if sodium is a problem for you) in a 32-ounce (quart) canning jar. Fill the jar with boiling water, and let steep at room temperature until cool. Strain or decant the liquid and discard the grounds, and then put a lid on the jar and refrigerate. Drink 1 cup (8 ounces) of the tea 4 times per day. After 1–3 weeks, drop to 1–2 cups per day or use as needed. For those with Type I diabetes, start with only 1–2 cups per day and increase by 1 cup per week, monitoring blood sugar closely. Buying cinnamon in bulk is cost-effective and highly recommended (see the Resources section).

Promising botanical treatments for Type II diabetes, based on animal studies include:

Common Name	Latin Binomial
Clove	*Syzygium aromaticum*
Cinnamon	*Cinnamomum spp.*
Bay leaf	*Laurus nobilis*
English walnut	*Juglans regia*
Juniper berries	*Juniperus communis*
Izui	*Polygonatum officinale*

Common Name	Latin Binomial
Syrian Christ thorn	*Zizyphus spina-christi*
Guduchi	*Tinospora cordifolia, T. crispa*
Cumin	*Cuminum cyminum*
Black cumin	*Nigella sativa*
Cucumber	*Cucumis sativus*
Bottle gourd	*Curcubita ficifolia*
Goat's rue	*Galega officinalis*
Reishi mushroom	*Ganoderma lucidum*
Java plum	*Syzygium jambolanum*
Siberian ginseng	*Eleutherococcus senticosus*
Coriander	*Coriandrum sativum*
Sage	*Salvia* spp.
Alfalfa	*Medicago sativa*
Bilberry	*Vaccinium myrtillus*
Damiana	*Turnera diffusa*

13

Natural Approaches for Preventing and Treating Diabetic Complications

Both Types I and II diabetes are associated with a number of potentially serious health conditions known as diabetic complications. Complications worsen with decreasing blood sugar control and increasing age and obesity. Diabetics who are nutrient deficient and who smoke tobacco or drink alcohol also have an increased risk for complications, including: increased risk for cardiovascular disease and stroke, poor circulation, difficulty walking or exercising, visual deterioration, and permanent, painful nerve damage.

If you have Type I diabetes, the irreversible nature of your condition means that you need to pay extra attention to preventing or minimizing complications. In almost all cases, complications eventually arise in Type I diabetes patients, but you can defer their onset for many years and minimize their impact on your health by controlling blood sugar, eating right, exercising, and starting on a supplement program as early in life as you can. This advice is especially relevant for parents with diabetic children. As a parent, you need to consider that your child may be facing a lifetime of insulin injections, and will never have the fine control of glucose metabolism that a nondiabetic child has. In order to ensure that your child can grow to adulthood as healthily as possible, you need to start supplementing *now*.

If you have Type II diabetes but don't have any serious complications, your first priority is to follow all the other suggestions in this book and try to reverse your condition. Your second priority is to follow the basic antioxidant supplementation in this section. Supplementation guidelines for *preventing* individual complications are also listed below. Please ask your doctor to candidly inform you of what complications you appear to be at greatest risk for developing, and choose your preventive supplements accordingly. If you have Type II diabetes and already have complications, please follow the supplementation guidelines for *treating* your complications accordingly.

If you don't have Type II diabetes but are at risk for it, follow the basic supplement plan in Chapter 8. This basic plan provides good protection for you. Preventing the eventual onset of Type II diabetes by getting started on the Modern Evolutionary Diet ensures that you need never suffer from diabetic complications.

Dr. Birdsall on Diabetic Complications

I asked Tim Birdsall, N.D., about diabetic complications. "I see cardiovascular complications the most, such as high trigylcerides, hypertension, elevated LDL cholesterol, and high total cholesterol," he said. "More severe complications such as neuropathy and retinopathy are mainly features of Type I diabetes. However, when Type II diabetes is allowed to progress to the point where insulin is required, the likelihood of developing severe or multiple complications greatly increases. In other words, the severity of the disease takes a big jump, and it also becomes much harder to treat. I start to see neuropathy and diabetic ulcers, for example, when insulin becomes required."

We both agreed that prevention with natural treatments and lifestyle changes is absolutely critical, at a *minimum,* to halt the progression of Type II diabetes before medications and especially insulin become necessary. We also both also agreed that ultimately Type II diabetes is reversible, as long as you start early and are willing to work hard.

Vitamin and Trace Mineral Antioxidants

Diabetics have higher levels of oxidative stress than nondiabetics. This is particularly true if blood sugar control is poor, but even if this is not the case, abnormal oxidative stress is still present to a significant degree. Exactly why this increased oxidative stress occurs is not known. It is likely due to a number of subtle metabolic changes brought on by diabetes, in addition to the gross change of abnormally high blood sugar. Regardless of the cause, it is important to recognize that increased oxidative stress is a major factor in all of the diabetic complications listed below. Equally important is the corollary that antioxidant supplementation is your first line of defense in preventing and treating all complications. This is one of the many reasons why the Modern Evolutionary Diet basic supplement plan includes antioxidant vitamins and trace elements. Following that plan is certainly beneficial; however, for preventing or reversing complications, the following slightly higher doses are recommended daily.

1,000 mg vitamin C with bioflavonoids 3–4 times per day
8,000 IU vitamin A
20,000 IU beta-carotene
100–200 mcg selenium
20 mg zinc, amino acid chelated or monomethionine
800 IU vitamin E, preferably as mixed natural tocopherols
200 mg alpha lipoic acid

Botanical Antioxidant Products

Botanical antioxidants are every bit as important as vitamin and mineral antioxidants. There are thousands of antioxidant phytochemicals in fruits, vegetables, and medicinal plants. These compounds are important on their own, and are synergistic with the vitamins and trace elements above. A basic principle of the Modern Evolutionary Diet is that since our ancestors routinely consumed a large variety of wild plants, we humans evolved literally "bathed" in phytochemicals. We have to consider that our good health depends in part on continuing this trend. We *need* to have green foods in our diet or we will never look or feel our best, nor fully prevent the onset of chronic diseases, including Type II diabetes.

The same applies for diabetic complications. Plenty of produce is a *must* for prevention and treatment of complications, as are the use of botanical antioxidant supplements. Some that are effective and widely available are listed below. Choose any 2–4 of these, and take 2 capsules twice per day. Switch or rotate products as you desire or your budget dictates. You may also find blends of antioxidants that make things easier, or traditional Chinese tonic/antioxidant blends that can be very beneficial. As a matter of fact, when it comes to antioxidant compounds in plants, they are the rule rather than the exception! Almost any blend of medicinal plants contains antioxidant phytochemicals; it is only a matter of how much, and what kind.

Any green drink (Many specifically advertise that they
   contain numerous botanical antioxidants.)
Curcumin (If you can afford only one, use this.)
Grape seed extract
Pine bark extract (Pycnogenol)
Licorice
Rosemary extract
Oregano, thyme, peppermint, spearmint, or other mint
   family plants, preferably as teas

Garlic
Cayenne
Siberian ginseng
Green tea beverage or extract
Mixed bioflavonoids
Mixed natural carotenoids
Schizandra

Specific Diabetic Complications

Supplementation guidelines for preventing and treating diabetic complications presume that you are taking antioxidants as well. The first few choices in each list are the most important, and are the ones to use if your budget or memory dictates how many supplements you can take every day. They are designated by a bullet.

In most cases, a single capsule of an herbal product is around 500 mg, so this dosage is often used in the following sections, and should be considered equivalent to one capsule or tablet, or one dose of a liquid extract. Occasionally a single capsule of a standardized extract or concentrated herbal product is less than 500 mg. If this is the case, follow the manufacturer's suggested dosage. When in doubt, using one capsule or tablet or dosage of an herb 3 times per day is almost always safe and usually effective. If this dose is too low, results may not be very rapid or obvious, and so you can increase by one capsule every 3–6 days, until you reach 6 per day.

Note: The following descriptions of complications are only brief outlines that explain the medical term for each condition. They are not intended to allow you to diagnose a complication yourself or for another person. They are also not intended to identify which complications you might be most at risk for. Please consult your physician for an individual, professional diagnosis, and then investigate which natural products may benefit you the most.

Neuropathy

Diabetic neuropathy is a progressive degeneration of nerve function, resulting in pain, tingling, and loss of sensation and muscle function. It is one of the most intractable and irreversible complications. It commonly affects peripheral nerves, that is, sensory and motor nerves going to places such as the hands and feet. However, all types of nerves can be affected. As the nerves degenerate, diabetics may feel tingling, burning, or pain and may have muscle wasting as well, since the nerves aren't stimulating the muscles correctly. Complete numbness or lack of sensation can occur.

The combination of diabetic neuropathy and angiopathy (damaged, blocked, and weakened blood vessels) is a causative factor for the very high incidence of impotence in diabetic men. It can affect men both physically and psychologically. These two diabetic complications can directly reduce blood circulation and nervous response in the groin and lower body in general. In some cases, diabetic neuropathy directly affects the nerves of the genitourinary system, causing impotence as well as urinary difficulties. In addition, the severe pain, burning, tingling, or numbness in the extremities caused by these conditions can cause emotional stress that inhibits a normal sex life.

One of the largest and most comprehensive human studies done on any natural product concerned the effect of gamma linolenic acid (GLA) on diabetic neuropathy. Two large multicenter clinical trials were conducted in which 202 diabetic patients were give 480 mg GLA per day for a year, and 202 other diabetic patients were given a vegetable oil placebo. In the group that received GLA, 25 of 28 parameters improved significantly. In the placebo group, 27 of 28 parameters showed deterioration. In the second year of the study, all patients were given GLA, and the 202 that were previously in the placebo group showed improvement instead of deterioration in 23 parameters.

Evening primrose oil, the source of GLA used in the study,

requires five or six 1,000 mg capsules per day to get the 480 mg GLA dosage. Evening primrose oil was used because of its greater effectiveness at improving nerve conduction velocity than borage oil or black currant seed oil. Diabetic neuropathy, of course, is a condition in which nerve conduction velocity (the speed at which nerve impulses travel) slows to below normal.

Alpha lipoic acid for diabetic neuropathy is another supplement studied fairly thoroughly in humans. In one double-blind placebo controlled study, 328 Type II diabetes patients were intravenously given 1,200, 600, or 100 mg alpha lipoic acid per day for 3 weeks. All doses significantly reduced pain and disability from neuropathy; however, the 600 mg dose was judged best, improving patients' symptoms 25 percent better than placebo. In other studies, doses of 400–900 mg per day were all shown to improve diabetic neuropathy and in times as short as 14 days. It must be noted that in many cases supplements were first given intravenously and then by mouth. An intravenous 500 mg supplement for 14 days was also shown to directly improve glucose utilization by 20–50 percent. A similar study with 600 mg by mouth for 30 days showed a trend toward increased energy metabolism, but the results were not as spectacular. Alpha lipoic acid is a fat-soluble antioxidant, as well as an enzyme cofactor used in energy metabolism, and so may play more than one role in preventing and treating diabetes. It appears best to take this supplement orally for some months in order to see maximum benefits.

In a 12-week randomized double-blind study of 24 patients, very high levels of B vitamins were found to significantly increase nerve conduction velocity. The patients received 8 capsules per day for 2 weeks, and then 3 capsules per day for 10 weeks. Each capsule contained 40 mg allithiamine (B_1), 90 mg B_6, and 250 mcg B_{12}, and so for the final 10 weeks they received 120 mg B_1, 270 mg B_6, and 750 mcg B_{12} per day.

Neuropathy Supplementation

- Evening primrose or borage oil. Preventive: 2–4 grams per day. Therapeutic: 5–7 grams per day.
- Alpha lipoic acid. Preventive: 200–400 mg per day. Therapeutic: 600–800 mg per day.
- Vitamin B_1. Preventive: 50 mg per day. Therapeutic: 100 mg per day.
- Vitamin B_6. Preventive: 50–75 mg per day. Therapeutic: 150–175 mg per day. Use higher doses only under professional advice or supervision.
- Vitamin B_{12}: Preventive: 50–200 mcg per day. Therapeutic: 500–1,000 mcg per day; in some cases injections may be necessary.

Also helpful:

Acetyl-L-carnitine. Preventive: 500 mg per day Therapeutic: 1–2 grams per day.
Chromium picolinate. Preventive: 400–600 mcg per day Therapeutic: 800–1,000 mcg per day.

This supplement has been shown to help reverse neuropathy, but this may be due to a substantial preexisiting chromium deficiency present in the individuals studied. Chromium picolinate is part of the most basic treatment for Type II diabetes and should be on your supplement list already.

Capsaicin (cayenne pepper extract): Used only as a topical preparation in the form of a cream to reduce painful neuropathy. Capsaicin cream has been proven effective for painful neuropathy, arthritis, and shingles in clinical studies.

Alpha Lipoic Acid and Evening Primrose Oil

David F. Horrobin, Ph.D., of Scotia Pharmaceuticals in the UK, said, "When alpha-lipoic acid is combined with evening primrose oil, there's about a thirtyfold increase in the effectiveness of both. This combination looks like it has tremendous potential for diabetic neuropathy. These observations are based on animal research, but more studies will definitely happen. It has both lipophilic (fat-soluble or fat-preferring) and hydrophilic (water-soluble or water-preferring) properties and links tocopherols (vitamin E), which can't get out of cell membranes, with ascorbates (vitamin C), which can't get into cell membranes."

This means that alpha lipoic acid may be important in the regeneration of antioxidants.

Retinopathy

Retinopathy is gradual visual deterioration caused by reduced circulation in the blood vessels that supply the retina. In response, and to increase the supply of blood to the eye, the body creates new blood vessels there. These new blood vessels are typically weak and fragile, and thus leak and cause serious hemorrhaging in the eyes. Diabetes may be characterized by high levels of the sugar sorbitol in the eye fluid, which can also contribute to retinopathy. Left unchecked, retinopathy can cause complete, irreversible blindness.

Anthocyanins and other flavonoids are the best approach known for treating this condition. For example, 60 Type II diabetes patients with diabetic retinopathy were randomly assigned to three treatment groups for 3 months: (1) o-beta-hyroxyethyl rutoside (brand name: Troxerutin; this is a form of the flavonoid rutin), 2 tablets per day; (2) butcher's broom extract, 2 tablets per day; or (3) pressed buckwheat, 6 tablets per day. At the beginning and on the last day of the study, each patient had a complete ophthalmological examination. Many patients had regression, not progression, of their disease with herbal treatment.

Blood glucose also decreased in all groups. Specifically, glycated hemoglobin decreased by 15.6 percent in the butcher's broom group and 3.3 percent in the buckwheat group, with less significant decreases in the Troxerutin group. The whole butcher's broom and buckwheat herbs were judged more effective than the Troxerutin alone. Butcher's broom and buckwheat definitely appeared to increase local blood circulation in the eye.

Bilberry is another anthocyanin-rich herb with a long history of use for improving vision. In one clinical study, 31 Type II diabetes patients were treated with standardized bilberry extract at 400 mg per day. All patients exhibited a reduced tendency toward capillary permeability and hemorrhaging, with the most improvements seen in the 20 patients who had diabetic retinopathy.

Retinopathy Supplementation

- Buckwheat. Preventive: 500 mg (or one capsule) 3 times per day. Therapeutic: 1,000 mg (or two capsules) 3 times per day.
- Butcher's broom. Preventive: 500 mg 2 times per day. Therapeutic: 1,000 mg 2–3 times per day.
- Bilberry. Preventive: 300–500 mg standardized herb per day. Therapeutic: 300–500 mg standardized herb 3 times per day.

Any one or all of these may also be helpful. Follow manufacturer's suggested dosage for tablets or capsules.

Ginkgo biloba
Bee pollen (a rich source of rutin): 2–4 tsp per day
Rutin (sometimes available as the individual bioflavonoid)
Proanthocyanidins (grape seed, pine bark extracts)

Cataracts

Cataracts are a progressive loss of transparency of the eye lens. The lens becomes grayish-white and somewhat opaque, resulting in blurred or distorted vision and an inability to handle glare. Untreated cataracts eventually cause complete blindness. Diabetics are prone to developing cataracts, especially at a relatively early age. This is due to high levels of glucose, and sorbitol or other sugar alcohols in the eye fluid, and a general increase in oxidative stress. For protection against cataracts, regardless of whether you are diabetic, the importance of aggressive antioxidant supplementation cannot be overemphasized. Certainly, smoking greatly increases your risk for cataracts as well. Quitting smoking is a must!

It is well known that vitamin A, which we synthesize from beta-carotene in our liver, is an essential element of the visual pigment in our eyes. The intact carotenoids lutein and zeaxanthin, however, are found in the macular pigment of our eyes to the exclusion of other carotenoids. This is an excellent example of how some phytochemicals should really be considered essential nutrients, because if our diet lacks these carotenoids, our vision directly suffers. Numerous epidemiological studies have shown that increased intake of antioxidant vitamins, fruits, vegetables, and carotenoids all reduce the risk for cataracts.

Taurine is the major free amino acid in the eye, and a deficiency may also play a role in the development of cataracts. In fact, deficiencies of many nutrients—including zinc, folic acid, other B vitamins, and vitamin D—are implicated in the development of cataracts. Although the incidence of cataracts increases greatly as we age, this may be due as much to poor nutrition (and smoking) as it is to aging. With a balanced nutrition supplement program and a diet with plenty of fruits and vegetables, we can treat cataracts naturally and even slow aging itself. Cataracts now affect 50 percent of the population over 75 years of age and are the *single largest line item* in the Medicare budget. Happily for us, though, the nutritional suggestions just given are the least costly and most practical means of reducing both the incidence and cost of cataracts and the treatment for them.

In a rat study, curcumin provided significant protection from cataract development induced by the oxidizing chemical

4-hydroxy-2-trans-nonenal (HNE) in rat eye lenses. The curcumin treatment not only protected against the damage done
by HNE, but also improved lens transparency over the control
situation—regardless of HNE damage or not.

Cataract Supplementation

The approach is mainly preventive. There is little evidence
that existing cataracts can be substantially reversed, but continuing damage may be prevented or slowed.

- Mixed natural carotenoid supplement including lutein,
  lycopene, and zeaxanthin: 10–20 mg per day
- Taurine: 500–1,000 mg per day
- Curcumin: 500 mg 3 times per day

Any one or all of these may also be helpful. Follow manufacturer's suggested dosage for tablets or capsules.

Alpha lipoic acid
Mixed bioflavonoids (rutin, quercetin, citrus peel extract)
Ginkgo
Bilberry
Schizandra
Rosemary and many mints

Microangiopathy, Peripheral Vascular Disease, Intermittent Claudication

Diabetic microangiopathy is a condition in which the smallest blood vessels thicken and stiffen. The circulation to these
small blood vessels is impaired, resulting in cold, numb, and
sometimes painful extremities. Peripheral vascular disease is a
more generalized impairment of circulation, which can affect
any blood vessel outside the heart and lymphatic system. It can
cause pain, numbness, fatigue, elevated blood pressure, and
skin pallor. In severe cases, areas of tissue may receive so little
blood that they become gangrenous and must be amputated.

Intermittent claudication is similar, but particularly affects the blood vessels that supply the legs. It is characterized by painful cramps in the calves and difficulty in walking a distance without pain. In all cases, smoking is a major cause of these conditions. If you smoke, you must stop to get better.

The combination of folic acid, B_6, and B_{12} helps prevent the excess accumulation of homocysteine in the body. Although homocysteine is a natural biochemical product of your metabolism, high homocysteine levels increase your risk for coronary heart disease, arteriosclerosis, and peripheral vascular disease among other conditions. Numerous epidemiological studies have correlated high homocysteine levels with greater risk for many cardiovascular and circulatory diseases and for pregnancy complications. In the basic supplement plan offered here, the levels of folic acid, B_6, and B_{12} are sufficient, especially since you should be taking them every day indefinitely.

For its part, L-carnitine is another supplement that improves pain-free walking and reduces general muscle pain in patients with intermittent claudication. Although disagreement does exist as to why L-carnitine is effective, it can be effective for a majority of those who suffer from these disorders, and is at least worth trying for 2 months or so to see if you benefit from it. If you do try L-carnitine, make sure you use 3–4 grams per day, as lower doses may not be effective. The downside is that L-carnitine is a very expensive supplement, and only a few suppliers have a high-quality product (see the Resources section).

Padma 28, an Ayurvedic blend of herbs, has also been shown repeatedly to improve the walking distance for patients with intermittent claudication.

Standardized extracts of ginkgo, *Centella asiatica*, bilberry, butcher's broom, mixed proanthocyanidins, and horse chestnut have all been found effective for peripheral vascular disease, microangiopathy, and venous insufficiency. They are especially effective for diabetics. Venous insufficiency is a condition characterized by generally poor venous circulation, especially in the lower legs. Varicose veins and chronically swollen ankles and feet are characteristic of milder forms of this condition.

Circulatory Disorders Supplementation

- Folic acid. Preventive: 400–600 mcg per day. Therapeutic: 600–1,000 mcg per day.
- Vitamin B_6. Preventive: 50–75 mg per day. Therapeutic: 100–150 mg per day.
- Vitamin B_{12}. Preventive: 100–200 mcg per day. Therapeutic: 500–800 mcg per day.
- Padma 28. Preventive: 1–2 tablets per day. Therapeutic: 4–6 tablets per day.
- L-carnitine. Preventive: 1–2 grams per day. Therapeutic: 3–4 grams per day.

In addition, any one to three of these at once is fine, or look for a blended product. Horse chestnut and butcher's broom are especially helpful for varicose veins and hemorrhoids. Use 3–4 capsules per day of each, unless otherwise directed by the manufacturer.

Gingko biloba
Horse chestnut
Bilberry
Gotu kola (*Centella asiatica*)
Butcher's broom

Any one or all of these may also be helpful. Follow manufacturer's suggested dosage for tablets or capsules.

Mixed proanthocyanidins (grape seed, pine bark extracts)
Garlic
Mixed bioflavonoids (rutin, quercetin, citrus peel extract)
Bee pollen: 2–4 teaspoons per day

Hyperlipidemia

Hyperlipidemia is a condition in which the blood plasma triglyceride (triacylglycerol) levels are abnormally high. Obesity, smoking, genetic factors, a high-fat (especially saturated and *trans*-fats) *and* high-calorie diet, excessive alcohol consumption, and liver dysfunction contribute to this condition, as does diabetes. I have selected herbal products that lower triglycerides and cholesterol and are also directly beneficial for glucose metabolism.

Fish oil, which is very effective at lowering triglycerides and many other risk factors for cardiovascular disease, is also safe for diabetics. High-dose niacin also has a long track record of lowering triglycerides and cholesterol, and is fairly often suggested by physicians. When using niacin, start with 100–200 mg with meals three times per day, and slowly increase the dosage, perhaps doubling it each week until achieving a desired level.

Another standarized extract of an herb used successfully in treating hyperlipidemia, this time in India, is guggul (*Commiphora wightii*), which in its gum resin form is sold as "gugulipid."

Let's also add fenugreek powder, which, in 100-gram doses in one study, lowered fasting glucose, LDL cholesterol, and triacyglycerols in Type I diabetes patients; 15–25 grams of fenugreek were similarly effective for Type II diabetes patients.

As for royal jelly, a very modest intake of 50–100 mg (dry weight) can reduce triglycerides by 10 percent and total cholesterol by 14 percent. This may be due to the high levels of pantothenic acid and sterols in royal jelly. Since royal jelly is a beneficial, nontoxic supplement that can be literally eaten as a food, it makes sense to give it a try.

Hyperlipidemia Supplementation

Generally, there is no need to supplement beyond the regular daily plan if you don't have this problem or if dietary changes alone are enough. However, the lower end of the dosage range or half the recommended dosage is an excellent choice if you think you are at risk for hyperlipidemia or just want to be prudent.

- Fish oil: 2–5 grams per day.
- Gugulipid: 500 mg 3 times per day.
- Fenugreek: 10–30 grams per day, or 5 grams standardized fiber product.
- Royal jelly: 500–1,000 mg (dry weight) per day.
- Niacin: 1.5–3 grams per day. Use under professional supervision only, and increase dosage slowly!
- Chromium picolinate: 400–800 mcg per day. Abnormally high triglycerides are a symptom of chromium deficiency. Chromium picolinate is part of the basic treatment for NIDDM, and should be on your supplement list already.

Any one to three of these at once is fine or look for blended products. Follow manufacturer's suggested dosage for herbs.

Boswellia
Garlic
Gurmar
Curcumin
Basil

Also helpful:

Flaxseed meal: 2 tbsp per day.
Flaxseed oil: doses of 2 tbsp or higher per day.
Panthothenic acid: 250–400 mg per day.

Hypercholesterolemia

Hypercholesterolemia is a condition in which blood plasma cholesterol is abnormally high. In addition, the ratio of LDL to HDL cholesterol is often higher than it should be. Obesity, smoking, genetic factors, excessive alcohol consumption, a high-fat *and* high-calorie diet, and liver dysfunction contribute to this condition, as does diabetes.

As discussed in the hyperlipidemia section, gugulipid, niacin, fenugreek, and royal jelly are all recommended for lowering cholesterol, as well as triglycerides. In addition to these treatments, beta-sitosterol and tocotrienols are two extremely safe natural products specifically for lowering cholesterol. These compounds are part of a larger groups of phytochemicals called phytosterols and isoprenoids, both of which can be fairly abundant in a diet that features large amounts of fresh produce, herbs, nuts, and unrefined vegetable oils. When oils are refined and processed, and plant foods consist mainly of refined cereal grains, these beneficial phytochemicals are lost from the diet. It's possible that this change alone plays a major role in today's epidemic of hypercholesterolemia.

Low-cholesterol or vegetarian diets can help to some degree, but are by no means panaceas. Often dietary cholesterol intake has little or no relation to blood cholesterol levels, and the increase in fruits, vegetables, and nuts in a vegetarian diet may be more important to the outcome than the decrease in cholesterol intake. It may be more important to: (1) maintain a high lean-to-fat body weight ratio; (2) eat a moderate-fat diet, with a balance of PUFA, MUFA, and SFA; and (3) eat plenty of plant foods and lean protein, and limit refined carbohydrates. A recent study showed, in fact, that simply replacing calories from sugar and starch with low-fat proteins such as turkey breast, cottage cheese, fish, and lean ham and beef reduced LDL cholesterol and triglycerides and raised HDL cholesterol in both normal and hypercholesterolemic subjects. This means that higher protein diets are both preventive and therapeutic for this condition. This should not surprise you by now, since it's just another reflection of how moving toward the Modern Evolutionary Diet protects us from chronic disease.

Hypercholesterolemia Supplementation

Generally, there is no need to supplement beyond the regular daily plan if you don't have this problem or if dietary changes alone are enough. However, the lower end of the dosage range or half the recommended dosage is an excellent choice if you think you are at risk for hypercholesterolemia or just want to be prudent.

- High-protein diet: Following the Modern Evolutionary Diet will take care of this.
- Tocotrienols: 150–300 mg per day.
- Gugulipid: 500 mg 3–4 times per day.
- Beta-sitosterol, alone or with mixed phytosterols: 4–6 grams per day.
- Royal jelly: 500–1,000 mg (dry weight) per day.
- Niacin: 1.5–3 grams per day. Use under professional supervision only, and increase dosage slowly!
- Chromium picolinate: 400–800 mcg per day. Abnormally high cholesterol and LDL-HDL ratios are symptoms of chromium deficiency. Chromium picolinate is part of the basic treatment for NIDDM, and should be on your supplement list already.

Any two or three of these at once is fine or look for blended products. Follow manufacturer's suggested dosage for herbs.

Boswellia
Garlic
Gurmar
Fenugreek
Curcumin
Basil

Also helpful:

Flaxseed meal: 2 tablespoons per day.
Oat bran: Use in meals as needed.
Panthothenic acid: 250–400 mg per day.

Abnormal Platelet Aggregation

This condition is an abnormal tendency for blood to clot or clump while still circulating in the blood vessels. Blood may be characterized as thicker than normal. Blood clots can lodge in veins or arteries, causing heart attacks, lung blockage, phlebitis, stroke, and other tissue damage. Blood clotting that occurs when you are cut or bruised, of course, is normal.

Fish oil is one of the most studied and effective natural products for inhibiting platelet aggregation. Although flaxseed oil does not lower triglycerides as effectively as does fish oil, it is effective at reducing platelet aggregation.

Curcumin was shown to inhibit platelet aggregation in a manner similar to aspirin; however, it is apparently safer. Low doses of aspirin inhibit platelet aggregation, but as the dosage increases, the effect becomes less and less beneficial. In contrast, curcumin becomes more beneficial as the dosage increases.

Taurine may be another nutrient that tends to be lower in diabetics. When 39 Type I diabetes patients were compared with 34 normal controls, it was found that the Type I diabetes patients had a greater tendency for platelets to aggregate, and lower levels of taurine. After supplementation with 1.5 grams taurine per day for 90 days, however, the Type I diabetes subjects' platelet aggregation improved to meet the mean value for the normal subjects. Taurine supplementation in the normal control subjects did not result in any further improvements in platelet aggregation, indicating that the diabetics were initially deficient in taurine.

Abnormal Aggregation Supplementation

Generally, there is no need to supplement beyond the regular daily plan if you don't have this problem. However, the lower end of the dosage range or half the recommended dosages is an excellent choice if you think you are at risk for abnormal platelet aggregation or just want to be prudent. Do not exceed lowest dosages *and* consult your physician first if you are already taking blood-thinning medication.

Fish oil: 2–5 grams per day.
Flaxseed oil: 4–6 teaspoons per day.
Curcumin: 500 mg 3 times per day.
Taurine: 1.5–2.5 grams per day.

Any one or two of these at once is fine, or look for blended products. Follow manufacturer's suggested dosage for herbs.

Garlic
Red clover
White willow
Aspirin: 1 baby tablet per day, or as recommended by a
    professional

Nephropathy

Diabetic nephropathy is a malfunction or reduced function of one or both kidneys. It results from damage to the capillaries that supply the kidneys with blood, as well as the network of tubules within the kidney that filter the blood. Nephropathy can be relatively minor and require only that you control your blood sugar and drink plenty of fluids, or it can be severe enough to require regular kidney dialysis. In general, nephropathy is considered to be a life-threatening condition, and is not very amenable to self-treatment. It is best to work with a physician who is holistically or nutritionally oriented to help you set up treatment that is individual to your case.

Throughout this book, I have indicated changes to my recommendations that apply if you have reduced kidney function. However, basic but not excessive vitamin, trace element, and antioxidant supplementation is still recommended, and in fact is considered necessary with severe nephropathy. The following other products can be beneficial, but in this case, ask your personal health care provider to set up a supplement program for you. Nephropathy is too individualized a condition to provide broad supplementation recommendations.

Fish oil

Taurine

L-carnitine

Folic acid (at levels of 1 mg or more per day)

Branched-chain and other specialized amino acid
supplements

Traditional Chinese medicine kidney herb blends—typically including rehmannia, lycium, atractolydes, aconite, alisma, hoelen, moutan, and other herbs. See the Resources section for appropriate product recommendations or consult a qualified traditional Chinese medicine practitioner.

An Interview with
Dr. Stephen C. Cunnane

Is Flaxseed a "Designer" Food?

Dr. Stephen C. Cunnane of the University of Toronto is an expert in the metabolism of PUFA in humans and animals. He has authored numerous publications in the lipids field. He has done considerable research on flaxseed products and LNA. I asked him first about the clinical benefits of flaxseed meal. He replied: "Aside from slowing down the absorption of carbohydrates, flaxseed meal is likely to reduce the clotting tendency of blood which may be abnormally elevated and this is a risk for vascular disease. This effect probably comes from the oil in flaxseed meal, which is rich in LNA, and surprisingly equivalent to fish n-3 fatty acids in reducing platelet aggregation. In comparison with what is published, flaxseed meal is similar in effect to comparable amounts of other types of soluble fiber, but carries the added benefit of being rich in a n-3 fatty acid, a relatively unique combination. I would definitely recommend that physicians try it, but if effects aren't satisfactory in amounts up to two ounces per day (about 60 g of flaxseed meal), it isn't worth trying more."

Stephen sees flaxseed meal as having potential to be a nutraceutical or "designer food": "I would fully agree with the 'designer food' potential of flaxseed meal; the niche markets of upscale bread bakeries and health food shops have clearly established its merits and acceptability. It will probably take the interest and financial commitment of a major company to help market flaxseed to its full potential.

Despite very positive research results and no safety issues at reasonable intakes (under 100 grams per day; higher doses haven't been tested), not many studies have been done, so the critical mass of peer-reviewed information is still low. This is partly due to a lack of funding targeting flaxseed, and partly due to the special precautions need- ed to keep flaxseed meal fresh once the packet is opened.

"Western diets are perilously close to being n-3 defi- cient, especially with such low fish consumption. The high intake of processed/hydrogenated oils and the low intake of green vegetables exacerbates this problem. I note that Dutch and French margarines have 2 to 5 percent LNA but this is not the case in North America, though clearly it is technically possible and acceptable to European con- sumers. Hence the persistant removal of LNA from seed oils (soybean, canola, etc.) is inexcusable and results in lower value products. The best reasons for including sup- plements of LNA in the diet are for reducing cancer risk and reducing abnormal blood clotting. LNA may have beneficial effects on the immune system but these are not well established or consistent at this time. Despite com- mon belief, LNA has no clear beneficial effects on blood lipids (i.e. triacylglycerols and cholesterol)."

I asked Dr. Cunnane to explain how a PUFA can be "conditionally essential"; that is, essential in some cases, but not in others. He replied: "Beyond the first few years of life, there is no evidence that DHA is strictly essential, but it is also very difficult to prove this because *healthy* adults have body stores (meaning storage fat) of LNA and DHA. It is true that there is slow conversion of LNA to DHA but this may increase if no DHA is consumed over long periods—it hasn't really be adequately studied.

"Weight loss and malnutrition *increase* the loss of LA and LNA from the body, and I personally believe LA and LNA have little importance in the body if the LC-PUFA are pre- sent in adequate amounts. Whether DHA is actually proven to be essential or conditionally essential is mostly

beside the point, because if you want to maintain optimal cardiovascular and mental health you won't go
wrong, and you'll probably do yourself a favor by regularly eating fish, which has pre-formed DHA. With
respect to AA, AA and DHA are better conserved by the
body than LA and LNA, which are easily oxidized for
energy. But AA will decrease if it isn't eaten, thereby
probably making it conditionally essential. However, the
same caveats apply from the discussion of DHA above."

Afterword

The food choices of past generations tend to be viewed later as outdated, unfashionable, and unhealthful. Each generation starts out fresh, redefining its cuisine and what foods constitute a healthful diet. My Great-Uncle Evans rose every morning before 5:00 A.M. to milk his cows and take the milk to the dairy. After these first of his many farm chores were done, he breakfasted heartily on eggs, bacon, scrapple, fresh creamy unpasteurized milk, homemade white bread toast with butter and jelly, and pie or cookies for "breakfast dessert." When I was a child, on winter Sunday nights after swimming practice, my mom fed us baked macaroni and cheese with slices of Polish sausage cooked right in the casserole. We had some salad also, and brownies with ice cream on top for dessert. These meals did the job for Evans and his son, and my brother and me, and were prepared with lots of love. Neither Evans' wife, my Aunt Edith, nor my mother thought for a moment that they might not be healthful.

Today, instead of my great-uncle's breakfast, we have 7-Eleven amaretto or French vanilla coffee supreme, fruit-flavored yogurt, and a whole wheat bagel, perhaps while driving to work. Macaroni and cheese homemade from scratch, considered both unhealthful and unstylish until recently, is back in fashion, thanks to low-fat cheese, soybean sausage, and the popularity of pasta. Today we indulge in a fat-free brownie and vanilla frozen yogurt instead of my childhood dessert.

When it comes to our nutritional requirements, however, none of the meals mentioned above are any more healthful than the other, and none of them are based on the foods that humans evolved eating. In order to define a healthful diet, we need to go back tens of thousands of years at least.

Although your body is still in the Stone Age, your mind and environment obviously are not. Most people cannot switch to the Modern Evolutionary Diet overnight. Be patient with yourself, but persistent. Also, keep in mind that your ancestors ate truly virgin organic foods. They were never exposed to agricultural products, let alone pesticides, herbicides, pollutants, medicated livestock, and highly processed foods. If you have a choice, try to help your health even more by consuming wild game and fish, free-range meats and eggs, and organic produce and dairy products. You will be pleasantly surprised at the superior taste.

It's not true that there can't be one diet for everyone, because if we generally stick to our evolutionary food choices, we avoid most of the diseases, problems, and allergies incurred by the all-too-recent adoption of agriculture and food processing. It's just that today's diet must be flexible enough to appeal to a variety of people and economic situations. The Modern Evolutionary Diet is the framework for all human nutrition, and you can make it work, regardless of your particular needs and circumstances. Upon this framework, you paint your own canvas. You may not be able to consume dairy products, may not be able to give up chocolate, or may choose not to eat meat, but this doesn't alter your basic nutritional requirements. If you want to lose fat without losing muscle, this is the place to begin. If you want to prevent or control Type II diabetes as quickly and effectively as you can, you won't find anything better than the Modern Evolutionary Diet.

The most important piece of advice I can give you from my heart is to set a good example. You can't persuade your family members or friends to change their diet, exercise, and take supplements if they are not willing to. But you can smile and go about doing so yourself, and so can your children. As you get healthier, there's a good chance that those you'd like to help will come around to your way of thinking. Sometimes their motivation is only jealousy, but more often it stems from love and respect—and a genuine desire to do whatever it takes to live a life free of diabetes!

Resources

Products, Services, and Further Information

The companies and products listed in this appendix are exactly the suppliers that I have used and continue to use in designing, fine-tuning, and putting the Modern Evolutionary Diet into practice. Therefore, I know that they offer products of high quality, or that are unique in the marketplace. If you choose to use these suppliers and manufacturers, I know that you can design a supplement/diet plan for yourself that will be effective. In most cases these companies offer reasonable prices also, but they are not usually the least expensive suppliers. In order to prevent or reverse NIDDM and treat IDDM it is necessary to have products that work, and that are backed up by the brand name guarantee of an honest company. The same is true of diagnostic testing such as blood food allergy tests, and the quality and taste of foods.

For the most reliable products, I recommend using health-food stores and mail order. I can't vouch for the quality or value of no-name discount products, multilevels, drug store, supermarket, and generic supplements, because I don't use them myself or in my practice. However, this is not a comprehensive listing of every applicable supplier in the natural products industry which offers these products, or which offers quality products. This is a large and rapidly growing industry, and undoubtedly you will find other products that you like, and more new supplements and designer foods targeted specifically towards diabetes will be coming on line in the next few years. So be open-minded and shop around, but use this Appendix, wholly or at least as a guide, to help you get started.

America's Finest

Piscataway, NJ 800-350-3305, www.afisupplements.com.
Ayurvedic herbs (*i.e.*, curcumin, gymnema, gugulipid)
probiotics
selenomethionine
specialty herbal formulations

Arizona Cactus Ranch

Green Valley, AZ 800-582-9903
prickly pear cactus (nopal) spreads and salsas

Aubrey Organics

Tampa, FL 800-282-7394, www.aubrey-organics.com
100% natural organic skin and hair prodcuts
   Your skin will benefit greatly from an "external" Evolutionary Diet containing natural herbs, proteins, and oils. If diabetes has caused you to have such problems as dry or scaly skin, skin rashes or itching, dandruff or drab hair, Aubrey has products that can *truly* heal your skin and scalp.

Beehive Botanicals, Inc.

Hayward, WI 800-233-4274, www.beehive-botanicals.com.
bee propolis, royal jelly, bee pollen, honey
specialty beehive products
natural skin, hair, and oral care products
   A good source for skin and hair care products featuring honey, royal jelly and propolis. These beehive ingredients can help heal problem skin. If you suffer from poor healing of cuts or diabetic ulcers, rinsing the area with propolis tincture in salt water, then using a salve featuring propolis can really help.

Biotics Research

Houston, TX 800-231-5777
oregano oil tablets
n-acetyl cysteine
specialty and professional supplements

Cactulife

Huntington Beach, CA 800-500-1713
encapsulated nopal

Carlson® Laboratories

Arlington Heights, IL 800-323-4141
E-Gems®
Key-E®
E-Sel
ADE®
   A superior line of Natural-Source Vitamin E, available in a variety of formulations, including soft gels, capsules, chewable tablets, drops, creams, ointments and spray.

CC Pollen

Phoenix, AZ 800-875-0096
High Desert® brand bee pollen, propolis, royal jelly, honey with royal jelly
oat, fruit and nut snack bars with bee pollen
specialty beehive products
   I eat only CC Pollen's pollen—I've never had any better, and I've been eating it for 15 years. Their whole line is the industry standard for quality, so don't settle for old, stale, dry pollen out of a bulk foods bin, or rancid royal jelly. My son loves the bars for snacks, and eats the orange chewable pollen wafers also. Ask for their Pet Power salve for healing wounds and ulcers.

Desert Essence, Inc.

Hauppauge, NY 800-645-5768 information only; sold in
health food stores and mail order catalogs.
Natural skin and hair care products
Tea tree oil and tee tree oil products
Natural toothpastes, mouthwashes, lip balms etc.

Tea tree oil used directly on the skin or nails is excellent for
getting rid of stubborn fungal infections. Use it also directly
on fresh wounds and to avoid developing infections and
ulcers. Tea tree oil shampoos are a good choice for dandruff
or for people with allergic skin and scalp problems. Dessert
Essence has a full line of (almost) 100% natural body care
products at reasonable prices.

Designs for Health Supplements

New Rochelle, NY 800-847-8302, www.dhfi.com.
L-Carnitine
alpha lipoic acid
specialty and professional supplements
custom-designed supplement plans

If you're going give L-carnitine a try, make sure you try a
brand name, such as the Lonza brand sold here. A good web
site to mention to a skeptical physician also, who might question your decision to use nutritional supplements. Designs for
Health can help you with a custom supplement plan if you're
interested.

Exercise Defined

Washington, DC 202-333-5227

Individualized instruction in Super Slow style weight training; Serious inquiries for Washington, DC metropolitan area
only. For information about Super Slow weight training in
your area, call the Super Slow Guild at 407-260-6204.

Experimental and Applied Sciences (EAS)

Golden, CO 800-923-4300, www.EAS.com
conjugated linoleic acid (CLA)
beta-hydroxy beta-methylbutyrate (HMB)
protein powder
Myoplex meal replacement drinks
Myoplex Plus Deluxe bars
alpha-lipoic acid
sports nutrition supplements
glutamine

While a whole foods diet is best, Myoplex powder in individual packages is a staple for me when I travel. Food is expensive in Europe and Japan, for example, and it can be hard to get large amounts of just plain protein without paying for an expensive dinner. Breakfast is really a problem everywhere, since it's often supplied "continental style" as pastries, breads, coffee, tea, and juice. This is a terrible way to start the day for diabetics and nondiabetics alike. Even restaurant breakfasts don't serve omelettes with 6 jumbo egg whites and two whole eggs, like I'd have at home. So a Myoplex mixed with milk and some flaxseed meal is a life saver. If I can't get milk, I use a few coffee creams and water.

Immuno Labs

Ft. Lauderdale, FL 800-231-9197 or 800-329-5991,
www.immunolabs.com.
microELISA blood food allergy testing
microELISA blood inhalant allergy testing
Candida antigen blood test
gluten sensitivity testing

Please ask for Kauley Jones and mention that you read about Immuno Labs in Dr. Broadhurst's book. If you choose to get food allergy testing, don't settle for inferior tests—they may be cheaper, but you get what you pay for. In many cases these tests are covered by insurance. Ask for a physician referral in your area if you need one.

East Earth Herbs

Eugene, OR 800-827-4372, www.eastearth.com.
Also sold in health food stores and selected mail order catalogs
Jade Chinese Herbals brand Chinese herbs
Stamina blend
Korean ginseng
herbal blends for improving kidney function

An accessible and inexpensive introduction to Chinese herbs; not overwhelming, and high quality is assured. In addition to the specific products mentioned in the text, the hay fever, cold and flu, insomnia, diet, and less stress products really work, but don't be afraid to increase the dosages listed on the bottle—they're fairly conservative.

Jarrow Formulas

Los Angeles, CA 800-726-0886
Information only; sold by health food stores and selected mail order catalogs.
large selection of vitamins, minerals, specialty supplements
sports nutrition supplements
glutamine
probiotics
garlic
acetyl-L-carnitine
CLA
alpha-lipoic acid
chromium picolinate

Jarrow can be counted on to provide high quality at a reasonable price, and to stay on the cutting edge of nutrition science. Jarrow-dophilus is an excellent probiotic, for example. Jarrow sells Omega Nutrition's Nutri-flax flaxseed meal and flax oils under his label also.

Kinakin International

Lnagley, BC Canada, 800-665-3908, www.RespirActin.com
RespirActin herbal liquid for improving respiratory function

RespirActin teas and lozenges

RespirActin is a one-of-kind product that is a big part of my natural treatment protocol for asthma. I've recommended it for those of you who have breathing problems or difficulty starting an exercise program, but give it a try if you're quitting smoking as well.

Nature's Herbs

American Fork, UT 800-437-2257, www.naturesherbs.com
Information only; sold by health food stores and selected mail order catalogs.
full line standardized herbal products
chromium picolinate
specialty supplements

Nature Sweet

St. Petersburg, FL 877-997-9338, www.sweetbalance.com
Sweet Balance Trutina Dulcem natural calorie-free sweetener
My favorite noncaloric sweetener by far, and can be used for baking and cooking.

Nature's Way

Springville, UT 800-962-8873, www.natureway.com.
Information only; sold by health food stores and selected mail order catalogs.
full line standardized herbal products
Efamol evening primrose oil
Efamol Efalex®
Neuromins® algal DHA supplements. This product is a more expensive source of DHA than fish oil, but is high quality, and suitable for vegetarians, young children, and those allergic to fish. For information about this supplement, go to the manufacturer's (Martek Biosciences, Columbia, MD) web site www.martekbio.com.
CLA
chromium picolinate
specialty supplements

Note: In Canada Efamol is distributed by Flora, Ltd. Burnaby, BC 604-436-6000.

Neways, Int.

Salem, UT 801-423-2800, www.neways.com.
Padma 28 formula (sold under name Badmaev 28)
Tibetan herbs
skin and hair care products

Next Nutrition

Carlsbad, CA 800-468-6398
Information only; sold by health food stores and selected mail order catalogs.
cold processed ion exchanged whey peptide protein powder
   There's many protein powders on the market, but you can't go wrong with Next Nutrition. The taste, mixability, and protein quality set an industry standard. Current flavors are vanilla praline, french vanilla, chocolate, strawberry and plain. If you've never used protein powder, start with a flavor, but as you grow to love it, the subtle taste of plain is really appreciated. Plain is also excellent for using in savory dishes, such as mixing with cottage cheese, sour cream, vegetable dips, or cooking with oatmeal. The strawberry is especially well done, and can convince anyone to eat a higher protein diet.

Nutrition Warehouse

Mineola, NY 800-645-2929, www.Nutrition-Warehouse.com.
   Discount mail order offering a full line of products from numerous suppliers, including TwinLab, Enzymatic Therapy, Nature's Herbs, Nature's Way, Jade Chinese Herbals, Country Life, Kyolic, Natrol, Next Nutrition, Jarrow Formulas, Source Naturals, and Nutrition Warehouse.

Ocean Nutrition Canada

Bedford, NS Canada, 888-980-8889, www.ocean-nutrition.com.
wide selection of pharmaceutical grade fish oil products
shark liver oil

fish oil combination supplements

We personally use Ocean Nutrition's fish oils at our home, and find it as pure and fresh tasting as any we've had. If you've had a bad fish oil experience, don't give up until you try these.

Omega Nutrition USA and Canada Ltd.

Bellingham, WA and Vancouver, BC Canada 800-661-3529, www.omegaflo.com.

PUFA supplements including flaxseed oil, Essential Balance™, and Essential Balance Jr.™

borage and evening primrose oil

organic coconut oil

other specialty cold-pressed oils

Nutri-Flax® organic flaxseed meal

probiotics

ayurvedic herbs

protein powder

glutamine

green drinks

garlic

stevia

alpha-lipoic acid

chromium picolinate

Neuromins® algae DHA supplements

specialty supplements (including Jarrow Formulas brand)

various other natural products, including skin and hair care

The only supplier of organic finely ground flaxmeal, which is a must-have for treating diabetes. Omega's oils are the ones I use at home and give as gifts. The quality is excellent, and all the oils are labeled with the pressing dates and expiration dates. You can get guaranteed fresh flax oil and Essential Balance oil by ordering directly from Omega. A good source for stevia and many of the supplements mentioned in the text as well.

Pacific Biologic Co.

Clayton, CA 800-869-8783, www.cyberforce.com/pacbio.
Padma 28 formula (sold under name Adaptrin)

Penzey's House of Spices

Muskego, WI 414-679-7207, www.penzeys.com.
bulk culinary herbs and spices (*i.e.*, fenugreek, cinnamon, garlic powder)
cocoa powder, baking extracts
salad dressing mixes

While I've recommended some specific herbs for diabetes treatment in the book, we've also noted that culinary herbs and spices are filled with antioxidants, and that it's a good idea to include more of them in your meals. Get a catalog from this company just on general principles—you won't be disappointed! They have hundreds of fresh high quality spices, herbs, and blends at great prices. You can buy a pound of cinnamon from Penzey's for the cost of two ounces in the grocery store, plus Penzey's has seven different kinds of cinnamon. I make sure I never run out of their Vietnamese cinnamon, Ceylon cinnamon, Maharajah curry powder, and Mexican oregano, among other products. They're the best I've ever tasted.

Sabinsa Corporation

Piscataway, NJ 732-777-1111, www.sabinsa.com
Information only; call for brand names in you local stores which include Sabinsa raw materials.
Ayurvedic herbs, including fenugreek, gymnema, curcumin, bitter melon, gugulipid, tinospora
Citrin®
BGOV vanadium complex
chromium picolinate
specialty supplements

Note that America's Finest, Health 2000, Neways, Nature's Herbs, Jarrow Formulas, TwinLab, Nature's Way, and others carry Sabinsa formulations. Sabinsa is the only manufacturer

I recommend for the standardized curcumin, bitter melon, and fenugreek fiber extracts mentioned in the book.

TwinLab

Ronkonkoma, NY 800-645-5626, www.twinlab.com.
Information only; sold by health food and drug stores and selected mail order catalogs.
full line nutritional, sports, specialty supplements, herbal blends

Almost any vitamin, mineral, or sport supplement mentioned in the text can be found under this label in a number of health food and drug stores. TwinLab has been in the business for a long time, and if you find yourself confused at the hundreds of bottles on the shelves of a vitamin "Superstore", you can't go wrong with TwinLab or Jarrow.

Worldwide Sport Nutrition

North Largo, FL 800-854-5019, www.sportnutrition.com
liquid protein syrup chocolate, peanut butter flavors
potassium pyruvate
protein powder
Pure Protein, High Performance, and Burn-It bars
Pure Protein fruit drinks and shakes in individual servings
sports nutrition supplements

When it comes to sports nutrition bars, it's hard to beat their Pure Protein bars. They have more protein in one bar than many vegetarians eat in two days. I keep the pure protein pina colada flavor drinks in my fridge for a quick 40 grams of protein on the run with no carbs or fat. A great snack for the Modern Evolutionary diet, and for diabetics. I also mix their chocolate or vanilla pure protein shakes 50/50 with whole milk and add some chocolate syrup to feed my 4 year old old son. I put in a bicycle bottle for him and shake. Much better than the overly sweet commercial chocolate milk, and no complaints at all. This "power chocolate milk" is a great idea for diabetics also, but you might want to use the "light" chocolate syrups or cocoa powder and stevia to sweeten it instead.

General Information

Chromium updates

For general information about chromium picolinate and chromium research, go to the manufacturer's website www.nutrition21.com. Manufacturer is Nutrition21, a division of AMBI, Inc., Purchase, NY.

High protein sports nutrition bars

The following bars are but a few of the many available that are higher protein, lower carbohydrate varieties. I have sampled over 100 bars, and the following choices are the ones that I recommend to others and purchase myself, and are the ones that were used in developing the Modern Evolutionary Diet. There are many worse bars, and few better.

These bars are all available in health food stores/supermarkets and becoming increasingly available in mainstream grocery and convenience stores. They come in a selection of different flavors, with chocolate, vanilla, fruit, and peanut butter the most common flavors. If you haven't tried these types of products yet, are making your first attempt to change a persistent candy bar habit, or are planning to give these bars to children, I recommend starting with Balance, Pure Protein, or PR*Ironman. The manufacturer is given after the bar name.

Keep in mind that these bars are not replacements for fresh whole foods and home cooked meals. All of these bars are trying as hard as they can to taste like candy, and many come very close. (Bars which are not high in protein sometimes come even closer, but I'm not even recommending these types here. Read the labels!) However, sports nutrition bars are much better choices than candy, bagels, muffins, and cookies, and are a good idea to help get you (or especially your children) on the road to eating a better diet. They make a good breakfast with coffee or tea if you're used to eating a donut, muffin, or cereal, for example. But don't overuse these products, or rely on them to keep feeding your sugar habit. If you become addicted to them, then you are still letting a sugar habit rule your life, regardless of whether or not you've given up your candy and pastries.

Balance Bar (Balance)
High Performance Bar (Worldwide Sport Nutrition)
Met-Rx Food Bar (Met-Rx)
Myoplex Plus Deluxe Bar (EAS)
PR* Ironman Bar (TwinLab)
Promax Bar (SportPharma)
Pure Protein (Worldwide Sport Nutrition)
Source One Bar (Met-Rx)

Suppliers of game meats, free range and/or all natural meat and fish products

Most of these are brands to look for in health food or gourmet supermarket, but some suppliers do sell directly, or will inform you of retail suppliers in your area. Many of these listed are precooked or prepared products. This is not because I think you shouldn't cook fresh food, but because I'd like to provide you with some alternatives to fast food and junky high carbohydrate prepared foods. If you've been mixing up boxes of macaroni and cheese, and microwaving pizzas, maybe you won't rush out to the fish market and buy a whole salmon to poach for lunch. But you might ease into a the Modern Evolutionary Diet by trying some all natural smoked salmon slices. There's no substitute for doing your own cooking, but 80% of good cooking comes from good ingredients. When you choose all natural free range meats, fish, eggs, and dairy products, you are choosing higher quality, better tasting ingredients that you will grow to love.

B3R Country Meats

West Childress, TX 940-937-3668 Natural beef.

Canadian Pure Farms

Chicago, IL 800-862-0060 Natural nitrate-free sausages.

Coleman Natural Products

Denver, CO 303-297-9393, www.colemannatural.com. Natural beef and deli items. The dei items are free of the many preservatives and fillers that typical deli meats have.

D'Artagnan

Jersey City, NJ 800-327-8246 Game meats and specialty meat and fish products. D'Artangnan has been supplying gourmet stores and restaurants with game meats for years. Now they're involved in the natural products industry because there is a rising demand for quality game meats and fish. If you don't hunt, here's where to buy venison and quail.

Fish Brothers Smoked Fish

Arcata, CA 800-244-0583, www.humbolt1.com/~fishbro/index.htm. Natural smoked fish. This company makes smoked fish like you would at home, with no preservatives or strange flavors. Even kids will eat it—try using it flaked like tuna salad.

Omega Foods

Eugene, OR 800-200-2356 All natural low fat salmon burgers. These come frozen in individual patty portions, which can be pan fried, baked, or carefully microwaved. They are an interesting and welcome alternative to canned tuna or sardines when you're in a hurry, but don't neglect using fresh fish in your diet. The company says they sell a lot to restaurants who use them in place of high-fat sausage in breakfast dishes, and they are indeed quite good along with eggs and hot sauce.

Royal Ostrich/Protos

Greensburg, PA 800-274-3263, www.protos-inc.com. Ostrich meat and ProTrim brand low fat ostrich meat sticks. Mail order source for fresh ostrich meat. The meat sticks are sold in health food and convenience stores, and do have nitrates, because it's required by law. However, they are a much healthier alternative to Slim Jims® etc, and are decent lean high protein snacks for when you're on the go. Unlike most mainstream cured meat products, they have a high ratio of potassium to sodium also. Older kids like them too, and don't seem to miss the fat at all.

Seaside Farms

Inglewood, CA 800-203-1500 Natural smoked and gravlax cured wild New Zealand Salmon, and Hawaiian smoked ahi tuna, ono, swordfish, mahi-mahi. Another company that smokes fish like you would at home, without preservatives. Wild salmon is hard to find these days, since most salmon is farm raised. Serve some of these products for a healthy holiday buffet, for example, and you'll find people who claim they don't like fish eating them right up.

Shelton's Poultry

Pomona, CA 909-623-4361, www.sheltons.com. Free range fresh poultry and prepared/ready to serve poultry products. Shelton is a leader in free-range poultry and their products are widely available. Be careful with some of their chicken franks, sausages, meatballs etc. as they are not low in fat.

SnackMasters

Ceres, CA 209-537-9770, www.snackmasters.com. Natural low fat beef, turkey, tuna, and salmon jerkies. Snackmasters has made nitrate-free jerky so widely available that I've even seen it next to the gummi bears and beer nuts in airport newsstands. A great choice when you're on the run, or to add a little bit of protein to your diet throughout the day. A small amount of jerky eaten slowly (it's hard to eat fast anyway!) is a great way to quell hunger pangs when dieting with very few calories.

Tallgrass Beef

Elmdale, KS 800-992-5967 Extra lean free-range beef.

Frontier Buffalo

New York, NY 888-EATBUFF, *www.eatbuff.com*. Lean buffalo meat that is range-raised and grass-fed with no hormones or antibiotics.

References

Chapter 1

Barakat HA et al. (1996). Lipoprotein metabolism in non-insulin-dependent diabetes mellitus. Journal of Nutritional Biochemistry 7, 586–598.

Broadhurst CL (1997a). Balanced intakes of natural triglycerides for optimum nutrition: an evolutionary and phytochemical perspective. Medical Hypotheses 49, 247–261.

Broadhurst CL (1997b). Nutrition and non-insulin dependent diabetes mellitus from an anthropological perspective. Alternative Medicine Review 2, 378–399.

Broadhurst CL et al. (1998). Rift Valley lake fish and shellfish provided brain-specific nutrition for early homo. British Journal of Nutrition 79, 3–21.

Bunn HT, Ezzo JA (1993). Hunting and scavenging by Plio-Pleistocene hominids: nutritional constraints, archeological patterns, and behavioral implications. Journal of Archeological Science 20, 365–398.

Carter JS et al. (1996). Non-insulin dependent diabetes mellitus in minorities in the United States. Annals of Internal Medicine 125, 221–232.

Cohen MN, Armelagos G (eds.) (1984). Paleopathology at the Origins of Agriculture. New York, NY: Academic Press.

Cooper RS et al. (1997). Prevalence of NIDDM among populations of the African diaspora. Diabetes Care 20, 343–348.

Crawford MA et al. (1970). Comparative studies on fatty acid composition of wild and domestic meats. International Journal of Biochemistry 1, 295–305.

Crawford MA (1992). The role of dietary fatty acids in biology: their place in the evolution of the human brain. Nutrition Reviews 50, 3–11.

Crawford MA, Marsh D (1995). Nutrition and Evolution. New Caanan, CT: Keats Publishing.

Eaton SB et al. (1997). Paleolithic nutrition revisited: a twelve-year retrospective on its nature and implications. European Journal of Clinical Nutrition 51, 207–216.

Elbein SC (1997). The genetics of human non-insulin dependent (Type 2) diabetes mellitus. Journal of Nutrition 127 (suppl.), 1891S–1986S.

Harris M, Ross EB (eds.) (1987). Food and Human Evolution. Philadelphia, PA: Temple University Press.

Harris SB et al. (1997). The prevalence of NIDDM and associated risk factors in Native Canadians. Diabetes Care 20, 185–187.

Howard BV et al. (1998). Relationships between insulin resistance and lipoproteins in nondiabetic African Americans, Hispanics, and Non-Hispanic Whites: the insulin resistance atherosclerosis study. Metabolism 47, 1174–1179.

Howard G et al. (1996). Insulin sensitivity and atherosclerosis. Circulation 93, 1809–1817.

Johns T (1996). Phytochemicals as evolutionary mediators of human nutritional physiology. International Journal of Pharmacognosy 34, 327–334.

Larsen CS (1995). Biological changes in populations with agriculture. Annual Reviews of Anthropology 4, 185–213.

Lillioja S et al. (1988). Insulin resistance as precursor of non-insulin dependent diabetes mellitus. Prospective studies of Pima Indians. New England Journal of Medicine 229, 1988–1992.

O'Dea K (1991). Traditional diet and food preferences of Australian Aboriginal hunter-gatherers. Philosophical Transactions of the Royal Society, London B 334, 233–241.

Sinclair A (1993). Was the hunter-gatherer diet prothrombotic? In: Sinclair A, Gibson R (eds.). Essential Fatty Acids and Eicosanoids: Invited Papers from the Third International

Conference, pp. 318–324. Champaign, IL: American Oil Chemists' Society Press.

Skelton RK, McHenry HM (1992). Evolutionary relationships among early hominids. Journal of Human Evolution 20, 493–503.

Speth JD (1989). Early hominid hunting and scavenging: the role of meat as an energy source. Journal of Human Evolution 18, 329–349.

Stewart KM (1994). Early hominid utilisation of fish resources and implications for seasonality and behavior. Journal of Human Evolution 27, 229–245.

Stringer CB (1992). Reconstructing recent human evolution. Philosophical Transactions of the Royal Society, London B 337, 217–241.

Suttles W (1968). Coping with abundance: subsistence on the Northwest coast. In: Lee RB, DeVore I (eds.). Man the Hunter, pp. 56–68. Chicago, IL: Aldine Publishing.

Szathmary EJE (1994). Non-insulin dependent diabetes mellitus among aboriginal North Americans. Annual Review of Anthropology 23, 457–482.

Tataranni PA et al. (1996). Role of lipids in development of non-insulin-dependent diabetes mellitus: lessons learned from Pima Indians. Lipids 31, S267–S270.

Tattersall I (1997). Out of Africa again . . . and again. Scientific American 276, 60–67.

Teufel NI (1996). Nutrient characteristics of southwest Native American pre-contact diets. Journal of Nutritional and Environmental Medicine 6, 273–284.

Chapter 2

Bjorntorp P (1991). Metabolic implications of body fat distribution. Diabetes Care 14, 1132–1143.

Branchtein L et al. (1997). Waist circumference and waist-to-hip ratio are related to gestational glucose tolerance. Diabetes Care 20, 509–511.

Flatt J-P (1995). Use and storage of carbohydrate and fat. American Journal of Clinical Nutrition 61 (suppl.), 952S–959S.

Gustafsson K et al. (1994). Dose-response effects of boiled carrots and effects of carrots in lactic acid in mixed meals on glycaemic response and satiety. European Journal of Clinical Nutrition 48, 386–396.

Jenkins DJA et al. (1981). Glycemic index of foods: a physiological basis for carbohydrate exchange. American Journal of Clinical Nutrition 34, 362–366.

Kissebah AH, Hennes MMI (1995). Central obesity and free fatty acid metabolism. Prostaglandins, Leukotrienes and Essential Fatty Acids 52, 209–211.

Macor C et al. (1997). Visceral adipose tissue impairs insulin secretion and insulin sensitivity but not energy expenditure in obesity. Metabolism 46, 123–129.

McKeigue PM et al. (1991). Relation of central obesity and insulin resistance with high diabetes prevalence and cardiovascular risk in South Asians. Lancet 337, 382–386.

Pi-Suyner FX (1996). Weight and non-insulin-dependent diabetes mellitus. American Journal of Clinical Nutrition 63 (suppl.), 426S–429S.

Shah M, Garg A (1996). High-fat and high-carbohydrate diets and energy balance. Diabetes Care 19, 1142–1152.

Truswell AS (1992). Glycaemic index of foods. European Journal of Clinical Nutrition 46 (suppl. 2), S91–S101.

Wolever TMS (1997). The glycemic index: flogging a dead horse? Diabetes Care 20, 452–456.

Chapter 3

Artal R et al. (1996). Exercise: an alternative therapy for gestational diabetes. The Physician and Sports Medicine 24, 54–66.

Calles-Escandon J et al. (1996). Exercise increases fat oxidation at rest unrelated to changes in energy balance or lipolysis. American Journal of Physiology 270, E1009–E1014.

Geliebter et al. (1997). Effects of strength or aerobic training on body composition, resting metabolic rate, and peak oxygen consumption in obese dieting subjects. American Journal of Clinical Nutrition 66, 557–563.

Ivy JL (1997). Role of exercise training in the prevention and treatment of insulin resistance and non-insulin-dependent diabetes mellitus. Sports Medicine 24, 321–336.

Lillioja S et al. (1987). Skeletal muscle capillary density and fiber type are possible determinants of in vivo insulin resistance in men. Journal of Clinical Investigation 80, 415–424.

Pan X-R et al. (1997). Effects of diet and exercise in preventing NIDDM in people with impaired glucose tolerance. Diabetes Care 20, 537–544.

Chapter 4

Anderson RA (1997). Nutritional factors influencing the glucose/insulin system: chromium. Journal of the American College of Nutrition 16, 404–410.

Anderson RA et al. (1992). Dietary chromium intake—freely chosen diets, institutional diets, and individual foods. Biological Trace Element Research 32, 117–121.

Anderson RA et al. (1996). Dietary chromium effects on tissue chromium concentrations and absorption in rats. Journal of Trace Elements in Experimental Medicine 9, 11–25.

Anderson RA et al. (1997). Elevated intakes of supplemental chromium improve glucose and insulin variables in individuals with Type 2 diabetes. Diabetes 46, 1786–1791.

Baynes KCR et al. (1997). Vitamin D, glucose tolerance and insulinemia in elderly men. Diabetologia 40, 344–347.

Blostein-Fujii A et al. (1997). Short term zinc supplementation in women with non-insulin-dependent diabetes mellitus: effects on plasma 5'-nucleotidase activities, insulin-like growth factor I concentrations, and lipoprotein oxidation rates in vitro. American Journal of Clinical Nutrition 66, 639–642.

Boden G et al. (1996). Effects of vanadyl sulfate on carbohydrate and lipid metabolism in patients with non-insulin-dependent diabetes mellitus. Metabolism 45, 1130–1135.

Broadhurst CL et al. (1997). Characterization by NMR and FTIR spectroscopy, and molecular modeling of chromium(III) picolinate and nicotinate complexes used for nutritional supplementation. Inorganic Biochemistry 66, 119–130.

Brun J-F et al. (1995). Effects of oral zinc gluconate on glucose effectiveness and insulin sensitivity in humans. Biological Trace Element Research 47, 385–391.

Capaldo B et al. (1991). Carnitine improves peripheral glucose disposal in non-insulin-dependent diabetic patients. Diabetes Research and Clinical Practice 14, 191–193.

Crayhon R (1998). The Carnitine Miracle. New York, NY: M. Evans and Co.

Eriksson J, Kohvakka A (1995). Magnesium and ascorbic acid supplementation in diabetes mellitus. Annals of Nutrition and Metabolism 39, 217–223.

Eibl NL et al. (1995). Hypomagnesemia in Type II diabetes: effect of a 3-month replacement therapy. Diabetes Care 18, 188–192.

Fairweather-Tait S, Hurrell RF (1996). Bioavailability of minerals and trace elements. Nutrition Research Reviews 9, 295–324.

Grimes DS (1996). Sunlight, cholesterol, and coronary heart disease. Quarterly Journal of Medicine 89, 579–589.

Halberstam M (1996). Oral vanadyl sulfate improves insulin sensitivity in NIDDM but not in obese nondiabetic subjects. Diabetes 45, 659–666.

Jovanovic-Peterson L, Peterson CM (1996). Vitamin and mineral deficiencies which may predispose to glucose intolerance of pregnancy. Journal of the American College of Nutrition 15, 14–20.

Liu J et al. (1997). Differential acute effects of oxovanadiums and insulin on glucose and lactate metabolism under in vivo and in vitro conditions. Metabolism 46, 562–572.

Oliveri MB et al. (1994). Serum levels of 25-hydroxyvitamin D in a year of residence on the Antarctic continent. European Journal of Clinical Nutrition 48, 397–401.

Paolisso G et al. (1993). Pharmacological doses of vitamin E improve insulin action in healthy subjects and non-insulin-dependent diabetic patients. American Journal of Clinical Nutrition 57, 650–656.

Pozzilli P et al. (1997). Vitamin E and nicotinamide have similar effects in maintaining residual beta cell function in recent onset insulin-dependent diabetes (the IMDIAB IV Study). European Journal of Endocrinology 137, 243–239.

Rogers KS, Mohan C (1994). Vitamin B_6 metabolism and diabetes. Biochemical Medicine and Metabolic Biology 52, 10–17.

Chapter 5

Ascherio A, Willett WC (1997). Health effects of *trans* fatty acids. American Journal of Clinical Nutrition 66 (suppl.), 1006S–1010S.

Borkman M et al. (1993). The relation between insulin sensitivity and the fatty acid composition of phospholipids in skeletal muscle. New England Journal of Medicine 328, 238–244.

Campbell LV et al. (1994). The high-monounsaturated fat diet as a practical alternative for NIDDM. Diabetes Care 17, 177–182.

Caughey GE et al. (1996). The effect on human tumor necrosis factor ∂ and interleukin 1ß production of diets enriched in n-3 fatty acids from vegetable oil or fish oil. American Journal of Clinical Nutrition 63, 116–122.

Chen Z-Y et al. (1995). Moderate, selective depletion of linoleate and ∂-linoleate in weight cycled rats. American Journal of Physiology 37, R498–R505.

Christiansen MD et al. (1997). Intake of a diet high in *trans* monounsaturated fatty acids or saturated fatty acids. Diabetes Care 20, 881–887.

Connor SL, Connor WE (1997). Are fish oils beneficial in the prevention and treatment of coronary artery disease? American Journal of Clinical Nutrition 66 (suppl.), 1020S–1031S.

Crawford MA (1993). The role of essential fatty acids in neural development: implications for perinatal nutrition. American Journal of Clinical Nutrition 57 (suppl.), 703S–710S.

Cunnane SC (1995). Metabolism and function of ∂-linolenic acid in humans. In: Cunnane SC, Thompson LU. Flaxseed in Human Nutrition, pp. 99–127. Champaign, IL: American Oil Chemists' Society Press.

Cunnane SC, Anderson MJ (1997). The majority of dietary linoelate in growing rats is ß-oxidized or stored in visceral fat. Journal of Nutrition 127, 146–152.

Das UN (1995). Essential fatty acid metabolism in patients with essential hypertension, diabetes mellitus and coronary heart disease. Prostaglandins, Leukotrienes and Essential Fatty Acids 52, 387–391.

Drevon CA et al. (eds.) (1993). Omega 3 Fatty Acids: Metabolism and Biological Effects. Basel: Birkhauser Verlag.

Dutta-Roy AK (1994). Insulin mediated processes in platelets, erythrocytes, and monocytes/macrophages: effects of essential fatty acid metabolism. Prostaglandins, Leukotrienes and Essential Fatty Acids 51, 385–399.

Gerster H (1998). Can adults adequately convert ∂-linolenic acid (18:3n–3) to eicosapentaenoic acid (20:5n–3) and docosahexaenoic acid (22:6n–3)? International Journal of Vitamin and Mineral Research 68, 159–173.

Harris CC et al. (1995). Mutagens from heated Chinese and US cooking oils. Journal of the National Cancer Institute 87, 836–841.

Harris WS (1997). N-3 fatty acids and serum lipoproteins: human studies. American Journal of Clinical Nutrition 65 (suppl.), 1645S–1654S.

Koletzko B, Braun M (1991). Arachidonic acid and early human growth: is there a relationship? Annals of Nutrition and Metabolism 35, 128–131.

Li D (1999). Effect of alpha-linoleic acid on thrombotic risk factors in vegetarians. Lipids, in press.

Luo J (1996). Dietary (n-3) polyunsaturated fatty acids improve adipocyte insulin action and glucose metabolism in insulin-resistant rats: relation to membrane fatty acids. Journal of Nutrition 126, 1951–1958.

Okuyama H et al. (1997). Dietary fatty acids—the n-6/n-3 balance and chronic elderly diseases. Excess linoleic acid and relative n-3 deficiency syndrome seen in Japan. Progress in Lipid Research 35, 409–457.

Pan DA et al. (1995). Skeletal muscle membrane lipid composition is related to adiposity and insulin action. Journal of Clinical Investigation 96, 2802–2808.

Pauletto P et al. (1996). Blood pressure, serum lipids, and fatty acids in populations on a lake-fish diet or on a vegetarian diet in Tanzania. Lipids 31, S309–S312.

Sarkkinen E et al. (1996). The effects of monounsaturated-fat enriched diet and polyunsaturated-fat enriched diet on lipid and glucose metabolism in subjects with impaired glucose tolerance. European Journal of Clinical Nutrition 60, 592–598.

Sinclair AJ et al. (1994). Diets rich in lean beef increase arachidonic acid and long-chain µ3 polyunsaturated fatty acid levels in plasma phospholipids. Lipids 29, 337–343.

Sirtori C et al. (1997). n-3 fatty acids do not lead to an increased diabetic risk in patients with hyperlipidemia and abnormal glucose tolerance. American Journal of Clinical Nutrition 65, 1874–1881.

Storlien LH et al. (1991). Influence of dietary fat composition on development of insulin resistance in rats. Diabetes 40, 280–289.

Storlien LH et al. (1996). Skeletal muscle membrane lipids and insulin resistance. Lipids 31, S262–S265.

Takahashi R et al. (1993). Evening primrose oil and fish oil in non-insulin-dependent diabetes. Prostaglandins, Leukotrienes and Essential Fatty Acids 49, 569–571.

Takeoka G et al. (1996). Volatile constituents of used frying oils. Journal of Agricultural and Food Chemistry 44, 654–660.

Chapter 6

Bressani R et al. (1983). Tannin in common beans: methods of analysis and effects on protein quality. Journal of Food Science 48, 1000–1001.

Cao G et al. (1996). Antioxidant capacity of tea and common vegetables. Journal of Agricultural and Food Chemistry 44, 3426–3431.

Crayhon R (1995). Robert Crayhon's Nutrition Made Simple. New York, NY: M. Evans and Co.

Daviglus ML et al. (1997). Fish consumption and the 30-year risk of fatal myocardial infarction. New England Journal of Medicine 336, 1046–1053.

Duke JA, Beckstrom-Sternberg S, Broadhurst CL. US Dept. of Agriculture Phytochemical and Ethnobotanical Data Base 1999: www.ars-grin.gov/duke.

Friedman M (1996). Nutritional value of proteins from different food sources. A review. Journal of Agricultural and Food Chemistry 44, 6–29.

Lemmon PWR (1997). Dietary protein requirements in athletes. Journal of Nutritional Biochemistry 8, 52–60.

Matsui T et al. (1997). Dietary skim milk powder increases ionized calcium in the small intestine of piglets compared to dietary defatted soybean flour. Journal of Nutrition 127, 1357–1361.

O'Dea K et al. (1990). Cholesterol lowering effect of a low fat diet containing lean beef is reversed by the addition of beef fat. American Journal of Clinical Nutrition 52, 491–494.

Sabate J et al. (1996). Nut consumption and coronary heart disease risk. In: Spiller GA (ed.). Handbook of Lipids in Human Nutrition, pp. 145–151. Boca Raton, FL: CRC Press.

Salmeron J et al. (1997). Dietary fiber, glycemic load, and risk of non-insulin dependent diabetes mellitus in women. Journal of the American Medical Association 77, 472–477.

Salmeron J et al. (1997). Dietary fiber, glycemic load, and risk of NIDDM in men. Diabetes Care 20, 545–550.

Scott LW et al. (1994). Effect of beef and chicken consumption on plasma lipid levels in hypercholesterolemic men. Archives of Internal Medicine 154, 1261–1267.

Srimal RC (1997). Turmeric: a brief review of medicinal properties. Fitoterapia 6, 483–493.

Thorogood M et al. (1994). Risk of death from cancer and ischemic heart disease in meat and non-meat eaters. British Medical Journal 308, 1667–1671.

Tuntawiroon M et al. (1991). Dose-dependent inhibitory effect of phenolic compounds in foods on nonheme-iron absorption in men. American Journal of Clinical Nutrition 53, 554–557.

Wang H et al. (1996). Total antioxidant capacity of fruits. Journal of Agricultural and Food Chemistry 44, 701–705.

Chapter 11

Ahmed T et al. (1997). Circulating antibodies to common food antigens in Japanese children with IDDM. Diabetes Care 20, 74–76.

Baur LA et al. (1998). The fatty acid composition of skeletal muscle membrane phospholipid: its relationship with the type of feeding and plasma glucose levels in young children. Metabolism 47, 106–112.

Braly J (1992). Dr. Braly's Food Allergy and Nutrition Revolution. New Canaan, CT: Keats Publishing.

Crook WG (1995). The Yeast Connection and the Woman. Jackson, TN: Professional Books.

Dosch H-M (1993). The possible link between insulin dependent (juvenile) diabetes mellitus and dietary cow milk. Clinical Biochemistry 26, 307–308.

Ellis TM, Atkinson MA (1996). Early infant diets and insulin-dependent diabetes. Lancet 347, 1464–1465.

Neu A et al. (1997). Incidence of IDDM in German children aged 0–14 years. Diabetes Care 20, 530–533.

Pettit DJ et al. (1997). Breastfeeding and incidence of non-insulin-dependent diabetes mellitus in Pima Indians. Lancet 350, 166–168.

Rensch MJ et al. (1996). Gluten-sensitive enteropathy in patients with insulin-dependent diabetes mellitus. Annals of Internal Medicine 124, 564–567.

Suresh B et al. (1997). Anticandidal activity of Santolina chamae-cyparissus volatile oil. Journal of Ethnopharmacology 55, 151–159.

Virtanen SM et al. (1994). Diet, cow's milk antibodies, and the risk of IDDM in Finnish children. Diabetologica 37, 381–387.

Chapter 12

Anderson RA et al. (1999). Isolation and characterization of chalcone polymers from cinnamon with insulin-like biological activity. Journal of Agriculture and Food Chemistry, in press.

Bailey CJ, Day C (1989). Traditional plant medicines as treatments for diabetes. Diabetes Care 12, 553–564.

Baskaran K et al. (1990). Antidiabetic effect of a leaf extract from *Gymnema sylvestre* in non-insulin-dependent diabetes mellitus patients. Journal of Ethnopharmacology 30, 295–305.

Bishayee A, Chatterjee M (1994). Hypolipidaemic and anti-atherosclerotic effects of oral *Gymnema sylvestre* R. Br. leaf extract in albino rats fed a high fat diet. Phytotherapy Research 8, 118–120.

Bordia A et al. (1997). Effect of ginger (*Zingiber officinale Rosc.*) and fenugreek (*Trigonella foenumgraecum L.*) on blood lipids, blood sugar, and platelet aggregation in patients with coronary artery disease. Prostaglandins Leukotrienes and Essential Fatty Acids 56, 379–384.

Broadhurst CL et al. (1999). Insulin-like biological activity of culinary and medicinal plant aqueous extracts. Journal of Agriculture and Food Chemistry, in press.

Cunnane SC et al. (1993). High ∂-linoleic flaxseed (*Linum usitatissimum*): some nutritional properties. British Journal of Nutrition 69, 443–453.

Frati AC et al. (1990). Hypoglycemic effect of *Opuntia ficus indica* in non-insulin-dependent diabetes mellitus patients. Phytotherapy Research 4, 195–197.

Head KA (1997). Type-I diabetes: prevention of the disease and its complications. Alternative Medicine Review 2, 256–281.

Koch H, Lawson L (1996). Garlic: The Science and Therapeutic Application of *Allium Sativum L.* and Related Species. Baltimore, MD: Williams & Wilkins Publishing.

Marles RJ, Farnsworth NR (1994). Plants as sources of antidiabetic agents. Economic and Medicinal Plant Research 6, 149–187.

Rai V et al. (1997). Effect of Ocimum sanctum leaf powder on blood lipoproteins, glycated proteins, and total amino acids in patients with non-insulin dependent diabetes mellitus. Journal of Nutritional and Environmental Medicine 7, 113–118.

Raman A, Lau A (1996). Anti-diabetic properties and phytochemistry of *Momordica chantaria L.* (Curcubitacea). Phytomedicine 2, 349–362.

Sharma RD et al. (1990). Effect of fenugreek seeds on blood glucose and serum lipids in type I diabetes. European Journal of Clinical Nutrition 44, 301–306.

Sharma RD et al. (1996). Hypolipidaemic effect of fenugreek seeds: a chronic study in non-insulin dependent diabetic patients. Phytotherapy Research 10, 332–334.

Sotaniemi EA et al. (1995). Ginseng therapy in non-insulin-dependent diabetic patients. Diabetes Care 18, 1373–1375.

Srivastava Y et al. (1993). Antidiabetic and adaptogenic properties of *Momordica charantia* extract: an experimental and clinical evaluation. Phytotherapy Research 7, 285–289.

Trejo-Gonzales A et al. (1996). A purified extract from prickly pear cactus (*Opuntia fulignosa*) controls experimentally induced diabetes in rats. Journal of Ethnopharmacology 55, 27–33.

Chapter 13

Archimowicz-Cyrylowska B et al. (1996). Clinical effect of buckwheat herb, *Ruscus* extract, and troxerutin on retinopathy and lipids in diabetic patients. Phytotherapy Research 10, 659–662.

Adler AJ, Holub BJ (1997). Effect of garlic and fish-oil supplementation on serum lipid and lipoprotein concentrations in hypercholesterolemic men. American Journal of Clinical Nutrition 65, 445–450.

Awasthi S et al. (1996). Curcumin protects against 4-hydroxy-2-trans-nonenal-induced cataract formation in rat lenses. American Journal of Clinical Nutrition 64, 761–766.

Brevetti G et al. (1988). Increases in walking distance in patients with peripheral vascular disease treated with L-carnitine: a double-blind cross-over study. Circulation 77, 767–773.

Brown WV (1995). Niacin for lipid disorders: indications, effectiveness and safety. Postgraduate Medicine 98, 185–193.

Cameron NE et al. (1998). Effects of alpha-lipoic acid on neurovascular function in diabetic rats: Interaction with essential fatty acids. Diabetologia 41, 390-99.

Ceriello A et al. (1991). Vitamin E reduction of protein glycosylation in diabetes: new prospect for prevention of diabetic complications? Diabetes Care 14, 68–72.

Dhawan BN (1996). A standardized Commiphora wighttii preparation for management of hyperlipidemic disorders. In: Balick

MJ et al. (eds). Medicinal Resources of the Tropical Forest. Biodiversity and Its Importance to Human Health, pp. 279–283. New York, NY: Columbia University Press.

Diehm C et al. (1996). Horse-chestnut seed extract: an option for treating edema. Lancet 347, 292–294.

Dines KC et al. (1996). Effectiveness of natural oils as sources of γ-linolenic acid to correct peripheral nerve conduction velocity abnormalities in diabetic rats: modulation by thromboxane A2 inhibition. Prostaglandins. Leukotrienes and Essential Fatty Acids 55, 159–165.

Franconi F (1995). Plasma and platelet taurine are reduced in subjects with insulin-dependent diabetes mellitus: effects of taurine supplementation. American Journal of Clinical Nutrition 61, 1115–1119.

Griesmacher A et al. (1995). Enhanced serum levels of thiobarbituric-acid-reactive substances in diabetes mellitus. American Journal of Medicine 98, 469–475.

Horrobin DF (1997). Essential fatty acids in the management of impaired nerve function in diabetes. Diabetes 46 (suppl.2), S90–S93.

Jacques PF et al. (1997). Long-term vitamin C supplement use and prevalence of early age-related lens opacities. American Journal of Clinical Nutrition 66, 911–916.

Jain SK et al. (1996). Effect of modest vitamin E supplementation on blood glycated hemoglobin and triglyceride levels and red cell indices in Type I diabetic patients. Journal of the American College of Nutrition 15, 458–461.

Miller AL, Kelly GS (1997). Homocysteine metabolism: nutritional modulation and impact on health and disease. Alternative Medicine Review 2, 234–254.

Qureshi AA et al. (1997). Novel tocotrienols of rice bran modulate cardiovascular disease risk parameters of hypercholesterolemic humans. Journal of Nutritional Biochemistry 8, 290–298.

Richter WO et al. (1996). Treatment of severe hypercholesterolemia with a combination of beta-sitosterol and lovastatin. Current Therapeutic Research 57, 497–505.

Rodrigues B et al. (1988). Effect of L-carnitine treatment on lipid metabolism and cardiac performance in chronically diabetic rats. Diabetes 37, 1358–1364.

Seddon J et al. (1996). A prospective study of cigarette smoking and age-related macular degeneration in women. Journal of the American Medical Association 276, 1141–1146.

Shimakawa T et al. (1997). Vitamin intake: a possible determination of plasma homocyst(e)ine among middle-aged adults. Annals of Epidemiology 7, 285–293.

Smulski HS et al. (1995). Placebo-controlled, double blind trial to determine the efficacy of the Tibetan plant preparation Padma 28 for intermittent claudication. Alternative Therapies in Health and Medicine 1, 44–49.

Snodderly DM (1995). Evidence for protection against age-related macular degeneration by carotenoids and antioxidant vitamins. American Journal of Clinical Nutrition 62 (suppl), 1448S–1461S.

Solzbach U et al. (1997). Vitamin C improves endothelial dysfunction of epicardial coronary arteries in hypertensive patients. Circulation 96, 1513–1519.

Srivastava KC et al. (1995). Curcumin, a major component of food spice turmeric (Curcuma longa) inhibits aggregation and alters eicosanoid metabolism in human blood platelets. Prostaglandins, Leukotrienes and Essential Fatty Acids 52, 223–227.

Stracke et al. (1996). A benfotiamine-vitamin B combination in the treatment of diabetic polyneuropathy. Experimental and Clinical Endocrinology and Diabetes 104, 311–316.

Yaqub BA et al. (1992). Effects of methylcobalamin on diabetic neuropathy. Clinical Neurology and Neurosurgery 94, 105–111.

Zeigler D, Gries FA (1997). ∂-lipoic acid in the treatment of diabetic peripheral and autonomic neuropathy. Diabetes 46 (suppl. 2), S62–S66.

Metric Conversion Charts

Formulas for conversion
Fahrenheit to Celsius: subtract 32, multiply by 5, then divide by 9
  for example:

$$212°F - 32 = 180$$
$$180 \times 5 = 900$$
$$900 \div 9 = 100°C$$

Celsius to Fahrenheit: multiply by 9, the divide by 5, then add 32
  for example:

$$100°C \times 9 = 900$$
$$900 \div 5 = 180$$
$$180 + 32 = 212°F$$

Temperatures (Fahrenheit to Celsius)

−10°F =	−23°C	coldest part of freezer
0°F =	−17°C	freezer
32°F =	0°C	water freezes
68°F =	20°C	room temperature
85°F =	29°C	
100°F =	38°C	
115°F =	46°C	water simmers
135°F =	57°C	water scalds
140°F =	60°C	
150°F =	66°C	

Temperatures (Fahrenheit to Celsius)

160°F = 71°C
170°F = 77°C
180°F = 82°C   water simmers
190°F = 88°C
200°F = 95°C
205°F = 96°C   water simmers
212°F = 100°C   water boils, at sea level
225°F = 110°C
250°F = 120°C   very low (or slow) oven
275°F = 135°C   very low (or slow) oven
300°F = 150°C   low (or slow) oven
325°F = 165°C   low (or moderately slow) oven
350°F = 180°C   moderate oven
375°F = 190°C   moderate (or moderately hot) oven
400°F = 205°C   hot oven
425°F = 220°C   hot oven
450°F = 230°C   very hot oven
475°F = 245°C   very hot oven
500°F = 260°C   extremely hot oven/broiling
525°F = 275°C   extremely hot oven/broiling

LIQUID MEASURES CONVERSION

For foods such as yogurt, applesauce, or cottage cheese that are not quite liquid, but not quite solid, use fluid measures for conversion.

Both systems, the US Standard and Metric, use spoon measures. The sizes are slightly different, but the difference is not significant in general cooking (It may, however, be significant in baking.)

Tbs = tablespoon   teas = teaspoon

Spoons, cups, pints, quarts	Fluid oz	Milliliters (ml), deciliters (dl) and liters (l); rounded off
1 teas	⅙ oz	5 ml
3 teas (1 Tbs)	½ oz	15 ml

Spoons, cups, pints, quarts	Fluid oz	Milliliters (ml), deciliters (dl) and liters (l); rounded off
1 Tbs	1 oz	¼ dl (or 1 Tbs)
4 Tbs (¼ c)	2 oz	½ dl (or 4 Tbs)
⅓ c	2⅔ oz	¾ dl
½ c	4 oz	1 dl
¾ c	6 oz	1¾ dl
1 c	8 oz	250 ml (or ¼ L)
2 c (1 pint)	16 oz	500 ml (or ½ L)
4 c (1 quart)	32 oz	1 L
4 qt (1 gallon)	128 oz	3¾ L

SOLID MEASURES CONVERSION

Converting solid measures between US standard and metrics is not as straightforward as it might seem. The density of the substance being measured makes a big difference in the volume to weight conversion. For example, 1 tablespoon of flour is ¼ ounce and 8.75 grams whereas 1 tablespoon of butter or shortening is ½ ounce and 15 grams. The following chart is intended as a guide only, some experimentation may be necessary to achieve success.

Formulas for conversion
ounces to grams: multiply ounces by 28.35
grams to ounces: multiply grams figure by .035

ounces	pounds	grams	kilograms
1		30	
4	¼	115	
8	½	225	
9		250	¼
12	¾	430	
16	1	450	
18		500	½
	2¼	1000	1
	5		2¼
	10		4½

LINEAR MEASURES CONVERSION

Pan sizes are very different in countries that use metrics versus the US standard. This is more significant in baking than in general cooking.

Formulas for conversion
   inches to centimeters: multiply the inch by 2.54
   centimeters to inches: multiply the centimeter by 0.39

inches	cm	inches	cm
½	1½	9	23
1	2½	10	25
2	5	12 (1 ft.)	30
3	8	14	35
4	10	15	38½
5	13	16	40
6	15	18	45
7	18	20	50
8	20	24 (2 ft.)	60

Index

abnormal platelet aggregation, 213–14
Acesulfame–K, 126
adult–onset diabetes, 21
aerobic exercise, 33–34, 35–36
aging, 21–22
  agriculture
  adoption of, 3
  changes with agriculture and food processing, 8–9
alkaloids, 178
alpha–linolenic acid (LNA), 73, 75–76, 78, 79
alpha lipoic acid, 54, 201, 202–3
American Diabetes Association Diet, 13
amino acids, 49
anaerobic exercise, 33, 34
anaphylactic shock, 163
anaphylaxis, 165
Anderson, Richard A., 51–53
angiopathy, 200
antioxidants, 62–63

botanical, 182, 198–99
vitamin and trace mineral, 197
arachidonic acid (AA), 73–74, 75, 76, 77, 78
artificial polyunsaturated fats, 69
aspartame, 126–27
asthma, 43, 161–62
Aubrey Organics Inc., 94–95
autoimmune diseases, 5
autoimmunity, 169
autosomal patterns, 12
Ayurvedic herbs, 191–92

B vitamins, 53, 54–55
Badmaev, Vladimir, 191–92
Beckman, Dennis, 40, 41
bee pollen, 111–12
beta–sitosterol, 211
bilberry, 54, 204
bioflavonoids, 125
Birdsall, Tim, 186–87, 196–97
birth control pills, 55